Managing Diversity and Inequality in Health Care

KT-103-341

Dedication

For my children:
Louisa, David, Neil and Martin

For Baillière Tindall:

Senior Commissioning Editor: Jacqueline Curthoys
Project Development Editor: Karen Gilmour
Project Manager: Jane Dingwall
Design Direction: George Ajayi

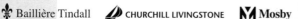

Six Steps to **Effective Management**

Managing Diversity and Inequality in Health Care

Edited by

Carol Baxter PhD MSc RGN RHV RM RN DN FETC HonFFPHM
Professor of Nursing, School of Health, Biological and Environmental
Sciences, Middlesex University, London, UK

Foreword by

Sir Alan Langlands
Principal and Vice Chancellor, University of Dundee, UK

Ba
PUBLI

EDINBURGH LON   ONTO 2001

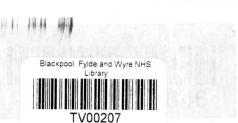

Baillière Tindall
An imprint of Harcourt Publishers Limited

© Harcourt Publishers Limited 2001

❦ is a registered trademark of Harcourt Publishers Limited

First published 2001

ISBN 0 7020 2520 8

British Library Cataloguing in Publication Data
A catalogue record for this book is available from the British Library

Library of Congress Cataloging in Publication Data
A catalog record for this book is available from the Library of Congress

Note
Medical knowledge is constantly changing. As new information becomes available, changes in treatment, procedures, equipment and the use of drugs become necessary. The editor, contributors and the publishers have taken care to ensure that the information given in this text is accurate and up to date. However, readers are strongly advised to confirm that the information, especially with regard to drug usage, complies with the latest legislation and standards of practice.

Printed in China

Six Steps to Effective Management series

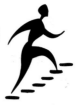

Managing the Business of Health Care
Edited by Julie Hyde and Frances Cooper

Managing and Implementing Decisions in Health Care
Edited by Ann Young and Mary Cooke

Managing and Leading Innovation in Health Care
Edited by Elizabeth Howkins and Cynthia Thornton

Managing Communication in Health Care
Edited by Mark Darley

Managing Diversity and Inequality in Health Care
Edited by Carol Baxter

Managing and Supporting People in Health Care
Edited by Margaret Buttigieg and Surrinder Kaur

Series editor: Ann Young

About the series
The Six Steps to Effective Management series comes at a time when the speed and extent of change within health care have rarely been greater, and the challenges facing nurses and everyone working within the health care sector are extensive. The series identifies and discusses those challenges and suggests ways of managing them. It aims to be unique in that it links theory with practice through the application of evidence where available and includes case studies which build on sound and relevant theoretical material.

All nurses are required by the clinical governance agenda to have a grasp of management principles. The *Six Steps to Effective Management* series is both practical enough to appeal to the practitioner and theoretical enough to be useful to those undertaking courses at undergraduate or diploma level. The books are relevant to all nurses.

The series comprises six volumes that are carefully constructed to contain a mix of theoretical and practical approaches, research and case studies, including a variety of perspectives from different sectors of health care. Each volume is relevant, realistic and practical to encourage reflection and critical thinking to prepare readers for flexible and adaptable styles of management.

For more information on this series please contact: Harcourt Health Sciences Health Professions Marketing Department on +44 20 7424 4200.

Contents

Contents

Contents

Contents

Contributors

Carol Baxter PhD MSc RGN RHV RM RN DN FETC HonFFPHM
Professor of Nursing, School of Health, Biological and
Environmental Sciences, Middlesex University, London

Barbara Burford MBAD Univ
Programme Director, Human Resources – NHS Employment,
Department of Health, Leeds

Lai Fong Chiu BA(Hons) MSc PhD CAES
Research/Clinical Effectiveness Co-ordinator, Wakefield and
Pontefract Community Health NHS Trust, Wakefield

Joy Foster BA PhD DASS CQSW
Principal Lecturer, Department of Education and Social
Sciences, University of Central Lancashire, Preston

Jennifer Harris PhD BA(Hons) CQSW
Senior Research Fellow, Social Policy Research Unit, University
of York, York

John James MSc
Director of Community and Specialist Services, Hounslow and
Spelthorne Community and Mental Health NHS Trust,
Hounslow, Middlesex

Martin Johnston BA MPhil
Senior Lecturer, Department of Health Studies, University of
Central Lancashire, Preston

Janet Knowles BSc MEd MSc CPsychol
Director, Knowldon Consultants Ltd, London

Irena Papadopoulos PhD MA(Ed) BA DipNEd DipN NDNCert RGN RM
Head of Research Centre for Transcultural Studies in Health,
School of Health, Biological and Environmental Sciences,
Middlesex University, London

Six Steps to **Effective Management**

Kelly Powell MB BS MRCGP MSc
Senior Registrar, Public Health Medicine, Merton, Sutton and Wandsworth NHS Health Authority, Mitcham, Surrey

Salman Rawaf PhD DCH DPH MPH MCH FFPHM FRCP
Director of Clinical Standards/Senior Lecturer, Merton, Sutton and Wandsworth NHS Health Authority, Mitcham, Surrey

Bob Sapey MA CQSW PGC
Lecturer in Applied Social Science, Lancaster University, Lancaster

John Stewart MA(Econ)
Senior Lecturer in Social Policy, Department of Applied Social Science, Lancaster University, Lancaster

Lesley Wade MA RGN CertEd
Recruitment Officer, School of Nursing, Midwifery and Health Visiting, University of Manchester, Manchester

Stephen Willcocks BA MA PhD
Principal Lecturer in Health Studies, Department of Health Studies, University of Central Lancashire, Preston

Application contributors

Jo Alleyne MSc (Nursing) BA(Hons) RN DipMgt(IM) MIMgt MIHM
Principal Lecturer, Nursing and Healthcare Management,
School of Health, Biological and Environmental Sciences,
Middlesex University, London

Sam Ayer RN BSc(Hons) PhD RNT FRSH
Senior Tutor, University of Hull, School of Nursing, Hull

Carol Baxter PhD MSc RGN RHV RM RN DN FETC HonFFPHM
Professor of Nursing, School of Health, Biological and
Environmental Sciences, Middlesex University, London

Louisa Baxter
At the time of writing this chapter, Louisa Baxter was a third
year medical student at Manchester University. Since 1998 she
has also been a member of Manchester Action on Street
Health – a voluntary agency which provides healthcare and
social support to female sex workers in the city.

Barbara Burford MBAD Univ
Programme Director, Human Resources – NHS Employment,
Department of Health, Leeds

Lai Fong Chiu BA(Hons) MSc PhD CAES
Research/Clinical Effectiveness Co-ordinator, Wakefield and
Pontefract Community Health NHS Trust, Wakefield

Christine Edwards BA MSc FCIPD
Head of Department of Human Resource Management,
Kingston University Business School, Kingston

Joy Foster BA PhD DASS CQSW
Principal Lecturer, Department of Education and Social
Sciences, University of Central Lancashire, Preston

Ann Gallagher RGN RMN BA(Hons) MA PGCEA
Research Assistant, Middlesex University, London

Pauline Ginnety RGN RM HV BA MSc PhD
Independent Consultant, Belfast

Six Steps to **Effective Management**

Sonia Harding SRN SCM HV BA(Hons) PGCE
Training and Development Manager, East London and the City
Mental Health Trust, St Clements Hospital, London; formerly
Positively Diverse Project Manager, Newham Community
Health Services NHS Trust, London

Jennifer Harris PhD BA(Hons) CQSW
Senior Research Fellow, Social Policy Research Unit, University
of York, York

Martin Johnston BA MPhil
Senior Lecturer, Department of Health Studies, University of
Central Lancashire, Preston

Mansour Jumaa RN FRSA FRSH DipNEd(Lond) BA(Hons) MSc MBA MA
Principal Lecturer, Health Care and Nursing Management; IM
Programme Director and Programme Leader, the MSc Clinical
Leadership Programme

Susan McLaren BSc PhD RGN
Professor of Nursing, Faculty of Health and Social Care
Sciences, Kingston University, Surrey

Tina Moore RGN Dip Nursing PGCEA BSc(Hons)
Senior Lecturer, Middlesex University, London

Olive Robinson BSc PhD
Industrial Fellow, Kingston University Business School, Kingston

Peter Ryan MSc CQSW
Head of Mental Health Training, School of Health, Biological
and Environmental Sciences, Middlesex University, London

Bob Sapey MA CQSW PGC
Lecturer in Applied Social Science, Lancaster University,
Lancaster

John Stewart MA(Econ)
Senior Lecturer in Social Policy, Department of Applied Social
Science, Lancaster University, Lancaster

Peter Toon MSc MRCGP AKC
Senior Lecturer in Primary Care, University College London

Margaret Whittock BSSc(Hons) PhD
Senior Researcher, Healthcare Management Research Centre,
Kingston University, Kingston

Dorothy Zack-Williams RGN RM RHV CPE BSc(Hons)
Health Visitor, Head of Inherited Blood Disorders, Abercromby
Health Centre, North Mersey Community NHS Trust, Liverpool

Application contributors

Foreword

The purpose of the UK National Health Service is to promote health, prevent ill health, diagnose and treat injury and disease and care for people with long-term health needs. The rights and services which flow from this purpose should be available to every citizen, regardless of gender, race, disability and age.

But, as the Government acknowledges in its recent NHS Plan, *the gap between health needs and health services remains stubbornly wide.* Tackling disadvantage and dealing with the fundamental causes of ill health is now the focus of cross-government action and a matter of real concern for vast numbers of NHS staff.

This volume, carefully edited by Carol Baxter, takes the question of diversity and inequality in health care head on. It reviews the relevant ethical and legal frameworks, provides many examples of good management practice and addresses critical questions of quality improvement in health care. Above all, it makes the case for the continued development of a diverse workforce, ensuring the effective and sensitive provision of services in a culturally diverse society.

Many nurses across the NHS prove day in and day out that they are first class leaders, breaking down barriers and making a real difference to the life opportunities and health of their local communities. It is my hope that the theoretical framework and the practical examples incorporated in this work will help them to achieve even more.

Dundee 2001   Sir Alan Langlands

Preface

> There is no such thing as a typical citizen. People's needs and concerns differ: between women and men for example, between the young and the old; and between those of different social, cultural and educational backgrounds and people with disabilities. Some of these concerns have not been given recognition in the past. We must understand the needs of people and respond to them. This too, is a crucial part of modernising government. (NHSE 2000)

This excerpt from the current government's equalities framework which provides national guidance for the NHS is the ideal epigraph for these prefacing words. That the differences and similarities which distinguish and unite us also challenge our intellect, emotions and skills in the workplace is increasingly being acknowledged. Developing competencies to manage diversity and inequality is particularly pertinent for nurses who provide care and support to people at their most vulnerable. Embracing this challenge and its accompanying enrichment is what this book is about.

The production of an edited volume is a long-term project (this one was over three years in the making). In reflecting on the developments which have taken place over this period, this preface outlines four inter-linking issues which are the main themes underpinning the book's contents:

- the emergence of a policy agenda
- a paradigm shift from goodwill to competence
- the link between employment practices and service delivery
- moving from the margins to mainstream of management.

THE EMERGENCE OF A POLICY AGENDA

Addressing the issue of equality has been intertwined with the interests of successive governments. There is a sense in which in the early 1990s, and leading up to the 1997 Health Service reforms, the concept of inequality came close to being abolished. For example, the first English health strategy, *The Health of the Nation* (HMSO 1992), was criticised for not acknowledging the structural component to ill health and the term 'inequalities' itself was notably replaced by 'social variation' in many government documents of that period. Now at the beginning of the twenty-first century it is fair to say that it has been rediscovered. Indeed over the last three years, as evidenced in the recent burgeoning of guidelines and policies, equality and fairness have become central themes of the NHS policy agenda.

This commitment is enshrined in the current government's modernisation strategy for the NHS (DoH 1997); the Independent Inquiry into inequalities in health (Acheson 1998); and *Saving Lives: Our healthier nation* (DoH 1999). These reforms have been followed by numerous other related developments including a progressive move away from a secondary to a primary care-led service, and a greater emphasis on improving management. A wider European dimension was subsequently introduced when the Human Rights Act of 1998, which sets out the rights of citizens to equal access to health care, came into effect in October 2000. These developments have conspired to bring the issue of managing diversity and equalities into greater prominence.

A PARIDIGM SHIFT FROM GOODWILL TO COMPETENCE

An important driver for change over the last few years is undoubtedly the fact that many groups in society are no longer prepared to tolerate gaps in health service provision and are becoming more effective at stating their case. For example, in relation to meeting the needs of patients with sickle cell disease (an inherited blood disorder with higher prevalence in ethnic minority communities), as far back as a decade ago, two health authorities made substantial out of court settlements to two families. Successful organisations are aware that it is not sufficient to be well intentioned: the familiar rhetoric of 'moral responsibility' is being replaced by recognition of legal and professional obligations. Awareness-raising training sessions which were popular in the eighties and early nineties are rapidly becoming a thing of the past. What is now considered good practice is emphasis on competencies and outcomes in relation to achieving organisational goals; best use of human and financial resources; and the taking of the strategic action required to bring about a paradigm shift from goodwill to competence.

THE LINK BETWEEN EMPLOYMENT PRACTICES AND SERVICE DELIVERY

Strategies to tackle inequalities in the past developed under the fallacy that the standard and nature of health care provided could be divorced from employment issues. Whilst a legislative framework of equal opportunities in employment has existed for some time, there was an absence of guidelines on equality in service delivery.

The recognition that the composition of the workforce is directly related to the quality of servicies to diverse clientele is now enshrined in the NHS Equalities Framework (NHSE 2000). This proposes an integrated approach to change underpinned by three strategic equality aims which are to:

- recruit, develop and retain a workforce that is able to deliver high quality services that are accessible, responsive and appropriate to meet the needs of different groups and individuals
- ensure that the NHS is a fair employer, achieving equality of opportunity and outcomes in the workplace
- ensure that the NHS uses its influence and resources as an employer to make a difference to the life opportunities and the health of its local community especially those who are shut out and disadvantaged.

MOVING FROM THE MARGINS TO MAINSTREAM OF MANAGEMENT

A number of developments have been indicative of the moving away of equality issues from the margins to centre stage. Firstly, increasingly the 'language of oppression' (characterised by reference to discrimination, prejudice, exclusion and marginalisation and the reciprocal strategies of anti-oppressive/ antiracism/antisexism) has given way to terms reflecting less confrontational and inclusive ideology: hence phrases such as

Pretace

'promotion of citizens' rights and responsibilities' and 'offering genuine choices for patients' are becoming a familiar part of the vocabulary. Associated with this trend is that of addressing the concerns of specific groups collectively rather than in isolation: the benefit of the former approach in addition to being less fragmented is taking the issues centre stage.

Whereas time-limited projects (not related to the main organisational priorities, funded from special monies and with little evaluation of outcomes) have characterised many initiatives to tackle inequalities in the NHS in recent years, those organisations which have made progress have come to appreciate the importance of a significant cultural shift towards the mainstreaming of these issues.

The NHS equalities framework which provides national guidance is an attempt to *equality proof* employment practice and service provision and then to *mainstream* equalities. Equality proofing involves placing equality considerations at the centre of decision-making and is a central element in the process of *mainstreaming* inequality. Mainstreaming goes beyond proofing in that it involves not only integration of an equality focus into policy but also the mobilisation of all policies behind the objective of achieving equality.

Another way in which the issues have been mainstreamed is through their association with change management. There is growing recognition that the further development of managerialism is compatible with and capable of providing for greater equality, equity, diversity and consumer involvement in service delivery. The prominence given to the role of leaders in bringing about change is also worth noting here.

OVERALL APPROACH

The aim of this volume is to raise the awareness of nurses and nurse managers about the issues of diversity and inequality and enable them to develop strategies to manage this at policy and practice levels. Ultimately, those wanting to bring about change must have several types of knowledge: knowing oneself; knowing the job; knowing the organisation; knowing the business; knowing the world. A leader must be able to perform certain core functions: valuing; coaching; empowering; team building and promoting quality. This book thus attempts to address all these issues.

Managing Diversity and Inequality in Health Care is designed both as a handbook and as a reader for use by individuals: the activities, tasks and reflection points may also be enriched through discussion with colleagues. Covering all common management problems, each of the 13 theoretical chapters provides key objectives, theoretical review of the subject matter, checklists and summary. Many of the practical applications are based on real life: it is hoped these will be familiar enough to enable readers to draw parallels with their own organisation both in the problems and solutions explored.

Managing Diversity and Inequality in Health Care aims to be both practical enough to appeal to the practitioner and theoretical enough to be useful to those undertaking courses at undergraduate or diploma level. It will not only support nurses who are new to their role but also those experienced nurses who wish to develop further. Nurses beginning a career in management or acting as equality advisors to Trusts or Health Authorities or managing specialist projects aimed at addressing inequalities should also find it useful.

This book is designed to enable the reader to:

- understand what is meant by diversity and inequality and the implications for managers in the NHS
- appreciate the ethical framework and legal imperatives which underpin responsibilities for workforce management
- explore the implications of strategic imperatives for managing a diverse workforce and issues of inequalities
- identify appropriate strategies for developing a diverse workforce to deliver care to culturally diverse clientele
- develop skills to meet the needs of diverse teams to address possible challenges
- recognise the benefits to service quality of a culturally competent workforce
- learn from the experiences of the private and independent sectors and from specialist services in the health and social care arenas.

In summary the new NHS has to think first and foremost about its patients, but also about multiple constituents such as societal values, labour markets, regulations and policies and technological advances. Nurse managers and their organisations will need to find workable, applicable ways of balancing these demands. This book is merely a start to what is undoubtedly a changing and developing field. We hope, however, that there is room for challenge and for creative problem solving. Ultimately nurse managers have to make their own way. We hope that this book will make some of those steps a little easier.

London 2001   Carol Baxter

References

Acheson D (Chair) 1998 Independent inquiry into inequalities in health report. Stationery Office, London

Department of Health 1997 The new NHS: modern and dependable. Stationery Office, London

Department of Health 1999 Saving lives: our healthier nation. DoH, London

HMSO 1992 The health of the nation. A strategy of health in England. Presented to Parliament by the Secretary of State for Health. HMSO, London

NHSE 2000 The vital connection. An equalities framework for the NHS. DoH, London

Section **One**

DIVERSITY AND INEQUALITY IN HEALTH CARE

Chapter Four   **87**
Researching women in primary care: the importance of the self in critical reflection
Lai Fong Chiu

Diversity and inequality in health care

Chapter **One**

Diversity and inequality in health and health care

Carol Baxter

OVERVIEW

A core principle of the government's plan for investment and reform in the NHS is the provision of services which are of high quality and are universal. Thus, services will be based on clinical need, comprehensive, patient centred, responsive to the different needs of different populations, able to reduce inequalities and support and value staff. As one of the largest groups of health service employees, nurses have a strong role to play in this process of change.

Six Steps to **Effective Management**

This chapter begins by identifying some of the demographic and wider societal trends which nurse managers are required to address in responding to the plural reality of Britain. The concept of managing diversity is defined with particular emphasis on its distinction from its precursor – equal opportunities. The term is critically examined and the benefits of managing diversity to the organisation discussed.

The second half of the chapter looks at inequalities in health and outlines the negative impact of socioeconomic group, ethnicity and gender on health status and access to services. The chapter concludes with a brief introduction and discussion of values clarification, cultural communication and leadership – essential skills in diversity competence.

INTRODUCTION

Throughout society mangers within organisations are increasingly being required to demonstrate competence in responding to demographic changes in the workforce, to ensure the efficient delivery of high-quality services based on evidence of effectiveness and to enhance customer service. These trends have brought about a refocusing on the way in which managers are developed, appraised and rewarded for their endeavours. The influence of these wider developments is reflected in the NHS, one of Europe's largest employers, and has particular relevance for nurses, its biggest group of employees. Some of the most fundamental changes affecting nursing are as follows.

- The fall in the supply of potential new recruits and high turnover rates of registered nurses.
- The increase in flexible working as a central aspect of NHS strategy to recruit and retain staff.
- An increase in the recruitment of nursing students and staff from overseas.
- The change in the balance of care between hospital and community and mergers with other institutional networks resulting in an increased diversity of the settings in which nurses work.
- Efforts to move care from expensive to cheaper health care providers has resulted in an increase in nurse-led services and the expansion of the nurse's role to include tasks traditionally carried out by doctors.

- Increasing recognition of the link between quality service delivery and quality management of staff.
- The recognition of need for more collaborative and interprofessional working and training in the NHS.
- The new roles and responsibilities of the nurse in supporting the government's modernisation agenda with its emphasis on improving public health and tackling inequalities.
- The move away from business orientation in health care management towards those with strong clinical backgrounds which has made the nurse manager a prime choice for promotion to senior management.

The demands on nurse managers in responding to diversity and change are thus now becoming more wide ranging and complex.

Based on material from two main sources (Acheson 1998, Kandola & Fullerton 1998), this chapter examines what is meant by managing diversity, outlines the nature of current inequalities in health and health care in the UK and discusses the implications of these for the development of nurse managers.

WHAT IS MEANT BY MANAGING DIVERSITY?

Demographic changes in the workforce

Over the last two decades the workforce within Western Europe has become increasingly diverse. The proportions of people from outside the traditional mainstream within the labour force have significantly increased and this is expected to continue for the foreseeable future (Ellison 1994). Despite this, their experience in the workplace is not the same as that of their counterparts (Box 1.1).

Cultural and social changes in society

At the same time as the demographic shifts there have been other changes in society influencing attitudes towards minority groups. A stronger lobby from minority groups for fair treatment has been particularly evident. Structural feminist critique, for example, has sought changes to work culture which would give a more positive view of part-time working, away from the notion of lack of ambition and towards increasing men's commitment to their domestic responsibilities.

Diversity and inequality in health care

Box 1.1 Inequalities in employment experiences

Ethnic minorities

- About 3 million people in Great Britain classify themselves as being from an ethnic minority group. This comprises 5.5% of the population.
- The ethnic minority population is on average younger than the white population (16% of the UK being over 65 years, whilst 3% of ethnic minority are within this age range).

- Economic activity rates are lower in the ethnic minority population: 74% black, 52% Pakistani and Bangladeshi and 80% white being economically active.
- Ethnic minorities are also more likely to be unemployed (18%) than their white counterparts (9%).

(Centre for Research in Ethnic Relations 1993)

Women

- Women are taking less time out of work to raise families and return in the interval between births.
- In 1997 women made up 44% of the labour force. It is expected that this will increase to 45.5% in 2001 and to 46% by 2006 (Ellison 1994).
- Well-qualified women are less likely to gain a job which reflects their qualifications than their male counterparts.
- Self-employment and part-time work have become flexible options for women to fit in with their domestic commitments.
- Women are overrepresented in service industries and non-manual occupations.
- Despite their increasing involvement in the labour market, many women still face barriers to entry into the labour force.

(Payne 1991)

Age

- There is a falling number of younger people entering the workforce, a phenomenon referred to in the UK as the demographic time bomb (Davidson 1991).
- It is estimated that the 16–25 year olds (a traditional source of labour) entering the labour market will have fallen by 1.5 million by 2000 (DoE 1988).
- Job applicants aged 55 or over are twice as likely to experience ageism than those between 32 and 38 years (37% and 16% respectively).

(This material is adapted from Diversity in Action *1998 Kandola R, Fullerton J with permission of the publisher, the Chartered Institute of Personnel and Development, CIPD House, Camp Road, London SW19 4UX)*

Box 1.1 Cont'd

Disability

● It is estimated that 6% of the labour force has a long-term health problem or disability.
● The employment rate for people with disabilities is 32% as compared with 77% for non-disabled people (Labour Force Survey 1997).
● A quarter of organisations do not meet the legal quota for employment of disabled people.
● More than half of employers expressed concern about disabled people's ability to do the job and their productivity; however, only a quarter of employers had experienced no difficulty (Honey et al 1993).

Carers

● About 7 million people (3 million men and 4 million women) in the UK spend some time regularly assisting an elderly relative or acquaintance.
● Approximately one in seven adults is a carer.
● Most carers are between 45 and 64 years old.
● About a quarter of carers spend 20 hours per week doing so.

(Berry-Lound 1993)

Gays and lesbians

● As a result of their sexual orientation, a fifth of gays and lesbians had experienced discrimination in applying for jobs.
● Eight per cent had been refused promotion and 4% dismissed.
● Over a half conceal their sexuality from colleagues.

(Equal Opportunities Review 1997)

An ethicolegal climate commensurate with the demographic changes has achieved more prominence in both public and private sector organisations. Ethics management is the implementation of an organisation's guiding values for creating an environment that supports ethically sound behaviour (Paine 1994). The European Union Code of Practice considers this issue from the viewpoint of the preservation of dignity at work. The matter of sexual harassment at work, for example, has been brought into sharper focus in recent years by a number of high-profile cases.

Many of these issues are covered by the antidiscrimination legislation which gives people the right not to be treated less favourably. Laws against sex, race, disability and age discrimination have been on the English statute books for some time. Within Europe, Britain and The Netherlands are at the forefront of legislation with regards to racial discrimination, whereas legisla-

Diversity and inequality in health and health care

tion protecting gays and lesbians is more firmly entrenched in France and The Netherlands. There are, however, growing trends towards both standardisation across Europe and a wider range of discriminatory grounds. The recent Employment Equality Bill 1997 in the Republic of Ireland now encompasses maternal status, family status, sexual orientation, religion and membership of the travelling community.

Managing diversity

Organisations throughout Europe now have to anticipate the implications of these changes for traditional working patterns and the subsequent impact on their policies and practices. Thus managing diversity begins with an acknowledgement of and planning for these trends.

The concept of diversity as a management tool has been around for some time. It has been particularly prominent in the literature relating to public sector organisations in the United States since the 1980s, rising to greater prominence with the emergence of the global economy and the growing degree of organisational flexibility and creativity which this warrants. In this context, the term has been subjected to several interpretations. It can mean integrating different parts of an organisation to enable them to work together (e.g. Calori 1988, Gold & Campbell 1987). It often also refers to matters of national culture within a multinational organisation (e.g. Bartlett & Ghoshal 1989, Phillips 1992, Trompena 1993). The most popular aspect of managing diversity, and one to which we subscribe, is its association with the advancement of equal opportunities.

A review carried out by Kandola & Fullerton (1998) covering both American and British literature during the 1980s and 1990s identified a number of definitions for managing diversity, several of which are included in Box 1.2.

There are very few divergences and an overall degree of consensus in these interpretations. Important features are:

- the wide range of differences encompassed: essentially, all ways in which people differ, not just the more obvious ones of gender, ethnicity and disability
- the premise that diversity and differences can add value to an organisation
- the organisational culture and the atmosphere within the workplace is of fundamental importance in the issue of diversity.

Essentially, then, managing diversity is the recognition that the workforce composition reflects people from a wide range

Diversity and inequality in health care

Box 1.2 Definitions of managing diversity (*This material is adapted from* Diversity in Action *1998 Kandola R, Fullerton J with permission of the publisher, the Chartered Institute of Personnel and Development, CIPD House, Comp Road, London SW19 4UX*)

Understanding that there are differences among employees and that these differences, if properly managed, are an asset to work being done more efficiently and effectively. Examples of diversity factors are: race, culture, ethnicity, gender, age, a disability, and work experience. (Bartz et al 1990, p 321)

People are different from one another in many ways – in age, gender, education, values, physical ability, mental capacity, personality, experiences, culture and the way each approaches work. Gaining the diversity advantage means acknowledging, understanding, and appreciating these differences and developing a workplace that enhances their value – by being flexible enough to meet needs and preferences – to create a motivating and rewarding environment. (Jameson & O'Mara 1991, pp 3–4)

Employers must 'seek out all available strategies that will bring them the talent they need to understand our own cultural filters and to accept differences in people so that each person is treated and valued as a unique individual'. (Kennedy & Everest 1991, p 50)

Managing diversity 'means enabling every member of your workforce to perform to his or her potential. It means getting from employees, first, everything we have a right to expect, and, second, if we do it well – everything they have to give'. (Thomas 1991, p 112)

The concept of managing diversity is inclusive – diversity includes white males. Managing diversity does not mean that white males are managing women and minorities, but rather that all managers are managing all employees. The objective becomes that of creating an environment that taps the potential of all employees without any group being advantaged by irrelevant classification or accident of birth. (Hammond & Kleiner 1992, p 7)

Diversity refers to much more than skin colour and gender. It can encompass age, race, religious affiliation, economic class, military experience and sexual orientation. (Galagan 1991, p 41)

of different backgrounds and experiences. Differences can be visible and obvious factors such as gender, race, ethnic group and disabilities through to less obvious factors such as religion, personality, work style and caring responsibilities. Capitalising on such differences will bring about a productive working

Diversity and inequality in health and health care

environment in which everyone feels appreciated and is empowered to fully use their talents to meet the goals of the organisation.

Moving on from equal opportunities

Equal opportunities have been promoted by organisations in both the public and private sector for the last 40 years. Whereas previously the emphasis was on aspects of discrimination and the legal obligations, in recent years organisations have come to appreciate that initiatives to address equality in the workplace stand a better chance of being sustained if they advance organisational goals and performance. For example, the arguments in relation to better maternity provisions and employment break opportunities for women are presented in terms of the potential to reduce the turnover rate of female employees. Similarly, arguing for the presence of people from minority ethnic communities and people who are disabled in the workforce is couched not merely in terms of fairness but in terms of the potential to gain access to a wider source of talent and develop closer links to a broader customer base. It is also argued that trust and commitment between employer and employees may result from ways of working which value staff and that business benefits will follow, such organisations show better overall financial performance, attract better staff, retain the best talent, benefit from lower absenteeism and demonstrate greater organisational flexibility to respond to change (Kandola & Fullerton 1998).

The following are the principal ways in which managing diversity differs from its precursor, equal opportunities.

Positive rather than defensive approach

There has been a tendency for equal opportunities policies to focus on the legal aspects and requirements to avoid discriminatory acts. Such a stance, in addition to being essentially defensive, can also limit initiatives to those areas which fall under the antidiscrimination legislation. Managing diversity, on the other hand, has a more positive message in relation to the overall organisational benefits of valuing and capitalising on the different backgrounds, characteristics and experiences of all employees.

Diversity and inequality in health care

Inclusive rather than exclusive

The traditional focus of equal opportunities on groups which are more systematically discriminated against in society can have the countereffect of creating resentment against such groups. Such a 'backlash' can occur when employees who do not fit into any of these categories begin to feel threatened or excluded. Managing diversity, however, adopts an inclusive approach, focusing on the individual rather than the group. This is less likely to engender feelings of alienation and more likely to gain the support of those within an organisation who have the power to promote policies and initiatives.

No special or unusual action

Equal opportunities relied heavily on the principle of positive action (allowed for under the various antidiscrimination legislation) where special measures such as training were undertaken to rectify the imbalances posed by social disadvantages. Positive (or affirmative) action runs the risk of being seen as positive discrimination in favour of particular groups. Such a perception, whether real or imagined, cannot be good for those 'not included' or for those viewed as 'reserved for special or preferential treatment'. Many women, black and ethnic minority and disabled people have felt 'set up' as a tokenistic gesture by organisations eager to prove they are equal opportunities employers. There is indeed an ongoing debate regarding the usefulness and sustainability of positive action and a call for it to be reviewed in the light of managing diversity.

The meeting of business objectives rather than head counting

The primary selling point of the effective management of diversity is its potential to help an organisation achieve its business objectives. Actions taken are therefore more likely to be evaluated to see if such outcomes have been achieved. For example, return rates of women after maternity leave, promotion ratios of groups who entered the organisation at the same time and access issues for people with a disability are all outcomes which can only be achieved if appropriate policies and systems are put into place. Managers need the right attitudes and skills to make this happen.

Diversity and inequality in health and health care

Hence managing diversity is about movement within and the culture of the organisation rather than merely counting up the number of new employees. It is about getting the best person for the job rather than appointing people because they are marginalised so everyone stands to gain and no one is 'set up to fail'.

Responsibility throughout the organisation

Traditionally, personnel and human resource departments have been responsible for equal opportunities. Managing diversity, however, sees responsibility as resting with everyone in the organisation, with managers having a leadership role. All managers are made accountable for the management of their staff and as such will need to be appropriately developed and supported to ensure they have the skills to manage a diverse workforce. Thus all managers have the potential to be high-quality practitioners in their own right.

The benefits of managing diversity

The overall benefits of managing diversity have been well articulated by its many protagonists (Cox & Blake 1990, Hall & Parker 1993, Hammond & Kleiner 1992, McEnrue 1993). Specific benefits such as 'unleashing energy from employees, freeing from the need to assimilate and play safe' (Hall & Parker 1993) and 'an enabling force for organisational change' (Ross & Schneider 1992) have been widely acclaimed although it is appreciated that many of the claims made will be difficult to prove or to encapsulate. Box 1.3 sets out the various levels of evidence as categorised by Kandola & Fullerton (1998).

Below we discuss two of the most frequently quoted benefits.

Access to and retention of talent and flexibility

Access to and retention of talent is one of the chief arguments for managing diversity. Reliance on the traditional pool of employees will inevitably limit access, since it ignores the remaining population and risks losing out to competitors. In a survey of organisations in Los Angeles, the majority of responding organisations gave attracting and retaining employees as their primary reason for introducing managing diversity (McEnrue 1993). Flexibility in terms and conditions is essential to meeting the individual needs of the workforce.

Diversity and inequality in health care

Box 1.3 Categorisation of perceived benefits of managing diversity (*This material is adapted from* Diversity in Action *1998 Kandola R, Fullerton J with permission of the publisher, the Chartered Institute of Personnel and Development, CIPD House, Comp Road, London SW19 4UX*)

Proven	*Access to talent* ● Making it easier to recruit scarce labour ● Recruiting from a wider range of talented candidates ● Retaining this talent ● Reducing costs associated with excessive turnover and absenteeism *Flexibility* Enhancing organisational flexibility
Debatable	*Teams* ● Promoting team creativity and innovation ● Improving problem solving ● Better decision making *Customers* ● Improving customer service ● Increasing sales to members of minority culture groups *Quality* Improving quality of services to customers
Indirect	*Staff gains* ● Satisfying work environments ● Improving morale and job satisfaction ● Improving relationships between different groups of workers *Organisational gains* ● Greater productivity ● Competitive edge ● Better public image

The introduction of flexible working practice by organisations has provided solid evidence of the benefits gained. Improved retention rates of women is among the most commonly cited. For example, Sainsbury's report that as a result of flexible working options the numbers of employees returning to work after maternity leave increased from 42% in 1989–90 to 74% in 1991–92 (Donaldson 1993). Reports from Boots reflect similar findings: their figures for shop assistants rose from 4% in 1989 to 49% in 1993 (New Ways to Work 1993).

Within the NHS, flexible working practices have been a major part of the strategy to resolve the labour shortage, the drive to

Diversity and inequality in health and health care

attract more people into the nursing profession and to encourage them back to the NHS resulting in a significant increase in the number of nurses working part time (DoH 1999a).

Associated organisational savings

The ensuing movement through the organisation to ensure the best people are the ones who advance and that individual talents are harnessed will result in cost effectiveness, particularly in relation to retention (Thomas 1991). A 1988 report by the Industrial Relations Service stated that one private sector organisation estimated their annual loss of 1000 women managers cost them £17 million every year (Syrett & Lammiman 1994). A recent Audit Commission Report (1997) identified that replacing a member of staff in the NHS can cost as much as £5000.

Some criticisms of managing diversity

Critics of managing diversity are far fewer than its proponents. One school of thought, based on a pragmatist perspective, suggests that the broad-brush approach to the various marginalised groups risks diffusing the very specific management effort required to challenge and change entrenched attitudes and practices. A rather more cynical viewpoint, associated with Lynch (1994), describes managing diversity as the

> new future oriented proportionalism that helps business harness this demographic destiny by exorcising the invisible demons of institutional racism/sexism and cleansing white male culture.

These two perspectives have largely been considered in our earlier discussions. With regard to the latter, however, it can be argued that the benefits of managing diversity should be assessed independently of the motivational factors behind it, whether they be self-seeking or altruistic.

INEQUALITIES IN HEALTH AND HEALTH CARE ACCESS

The nature of health inequalities

Most people would subscribe to the view that all individuals should have an equal and fair opportunity to enjoy life's benefits, including optimising their health status. However, inequalities occur as a consequence of differences in opportunities amongst individuals and groups. Deciding what is fair and just comes down to a subjective judgement in the end but many would probably agree with the comments on social justice expressed by the WHO (1985a) as follows.

> In health terms, 'ideally, everyone should have the same opportunity to attain the highest level of health and more pragmatically, none should be unduly disadvantaged'.

> In health care the principle of social justice 'leads to equal access to available care, equal treatment for equal access and equal quality of care'.

Health is taken to encompass physical, social and emotional well-being and is increasingly seen in terms of a positive resource for life rather than an objective of living (WHO 1978, 1984). Such a definition implies that the determinants of health are multidimensional and interrelated (Whitehead 1995). One acknowledged approach to classifying these multiple impacts on health is the health fields model (LaLonde 1974) (Fig. 1.1).

Human beings vary in health as they do in every other aspect of their lives. Biological factors such as age, sex and genotype have a major influence on health. Lifestyle factors are by definition those that the individual undertakes from his or her own choice and will include, for example, smoking habits and physical activity. Environmental influences in contrast are those over which the individual has little or no control and would include the quality of air

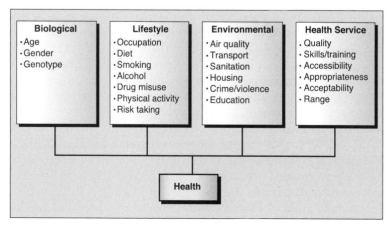

Figure 1.1 The Lalonde health field model (reproduced from Lalonde 1974)

and water. Health service factors include access to and uptake of appropriate health care.

A traditional way of determining inequalities is to document their existence in terms of:

- mortality (usually expressed as death rates and life expectancy)
- morbidity (usually expressed as limiting long-standing illness)
- access to appropriate health care services.

Current inequalities in health

In Britain, analysing national statistics to shed light on the nature and causes of social inequalities in health has gone on for the past 200 years (Whitehead 1997). Evidence on social inequalities and inadequate access to health care in Britain also played a key role in pressure to set up the welfare state in the postwar period, the landmark Beveridge Report (1942) being the blueprint for this.

Concern about persisting health inequalities in the 1970s led to the Black Report (Black et al 1980). This also influenced the decision of the member states of the European Region of the WHO (including the UK) to agree a common health strategy in 1985, with equity in health as a theme running right through it and reduction in inequities as the subject of the first of 38 targets to be achieved by the year 2000 (WHO 1985b). This report is viewed as one of the first comprehensive attempts by the government to explain trends in inequalities in health and relate these to policies intended to promote as well as restore health (Townsend et al 1992).

The Acheson Report (1998) summarises the current health trends, including expectation of life and inequalities for England and Wales. It identifies a number of variables that impact on health and concludes that an individual's chance of a long and healthy life is influenced predominantly by how well off they are, their ethnic group, gender and age. Where detrimental factors coexist (for example, unemployment, low pay and poor housing) their interaction leads to a disproportionate effect on health. Current health status, whilst improving for all socioeconomic groups, shows a widening gap between those at the top (professionals) and those at the bottom (manual workers). Uptake of and access to services show similar disparities between groups in society. In particular, the negative impact of socioeconomic group, ethnicity and gender has been demonstrated, the key aspects of which are outlined below.

Socioeconomic inequalities

- Over the last 25 years, there have been falls in death rates from a number of important causes of death, for example, lung cancer (for men only), coronary heart disease and stroke. However, the difference in rates between those at the top and bottom of the social scale has widened.
- Infant mortality rates are higher among babies born to families in social classes IV and V. The class differential had not fallen between 1994 and 1996.
- Premature mortality (that is, deaths before the age of 65) is higher among people who are unskilled.
- Death rates from major accidents and suicides among men are more common in the manual classes for those under age 55.
- Life expectancy has risen over the last century and is considerably higher among the higher social classes (75 and 70 years for men and 80 and 77 years for women in the higher and lower socioeconomic groups respectively).
- Higher rates of general practitioner consultation are associated with greater social and economic deprivation, even after adjusting for need.
- Communities most at risk of ill health tend to experience the least satisfactory access to the full range of preventive services, the so-called inverse prevention law.
- For outpatients, attendance is either higher in disadvantaged groups or similar to the better off, after adjusting for need.
- The use of psychiatric, especially inpatient hospital, services is positively correlated with high levels of deprivation and unemployment.

Ethnic inequalities

- Ethnic group is not yet routinely collected and so in analysing mortality rates, country of birth has to be used as a proxy for ethnicity.
- Perinatal mortality rates have been consistently higher for babies of mothers born outside the UK. The differences between groups have not decreased over the last 20 years.
- Among mothers who were born in countries outside the UK, those from the Caribbean and Pakistan have infant mortality rates about double the national average.
- There is excess mortality among men and women born in Africa, men born on the Indian subcontinent and men and women born in Scotland or Ireland.

Diversity and inequality in health and health care

- People in black (Caribbean, African and other) groups and Indians have higher rates of limiting long-standing illness than white people.
- For some minority ethnic groups, outpatient attendance rates are lower than for the ethnic majority.
- There is evidence of high inpatient admission rates for schizophrenia but lower consultation rates for mental health problems among young African Caribbean men.
- In contrast, women and men from South Asian populations have much lower rates of GP consultation for mental health problems than the white population.
- Differences in socioeconomic status do not account for differences in mortality between migrant groups.

Gender inequalities

- Death rates have been falling for both males and females. Since 1971, these have decreased by 29% for males and 25% for females, narrowing the differential in death rates very slightly.
- At each age in childhood and on into adulthood, the age-specific mortality rate for boys is higher than for girls.
- Cancers and coronary heart disease account for 55% of the deaths of men and 42% of the deaths of women.
- Healthy life expectancy of females is only 2–3 years more than that of males.
- For both children and adults of working ages, males have higher major accident rates than females. At older ages, women have higher major accident rates than men.
- The proportion of smokers is higher among girls than boys.
- Women tend to experience more long-term illness and disability.

Inequality in access to appropriate health care services

The relationship between access to services and inequalities is complex in that, as well as being an outcome, access to health care can also be a determinant of health status and subsequent inequalities. Factors in the way services are supplied, such as geographical distribution, the range and quality, timing and organisation of service, distance, availability of staff, their levels of training, education and recruitment, can all impact on uptake and whether people benefit from services. Similarly, demand factors, such as an individual's health beliefs and knowledge about available services, can determine whether they use services.

Health professionals may hold the same negative attitudes that are found in the rest of society. Lack of mutual understanding between them and service users can lead to negative perceptions which affect professional judgements and relationships. The resulting impact of this social distance on the treatment of traditionally devalued groups may thus be a contributory factor to inequalities in health care and health outcomes. Most nurses would not deliberately withhold care or treat people differently on the basis of their background. However, institutional discrimination within services is more pervasive and damaging and occurs in a variety of ways:

- by default where the ways in which things are done do not take account of the needs of a specific (usually minority) group
- health professional behaviour (whether conscious or unconscious) towards patients from different groups can be based on stereotyping and prejudice
- policies and practices within services can have the effect of excluding some groups whilst maintaining the privileged position of others.

Thus ambivalent attitudes towards and less favourable treatment of, for example, ethnic minorities (Baxter & Baxter 2000, Bowler 1993, Larbie 1984, McNaught 1985), disabled people (Bailey 1994, Brillhart et al 1990), gays and lesbians (Platzer 1993) and people with learning disabilities (Brown et al 1994, Turk & Brown 1992) have been identified in nursing practice. Such experiences can also act as a deterrent to service uptake by these sections of the population.

ADDRESSING DIVERSITY AND INEQUALITY IN THE DEVELOPMENT OF THE NURSE MANAGER

The management of change

The challenge for the health service in managing staff, patient and provider diversity issues is to plan effectively to ensure that it understands the health and health care needs of its diverse clientele and that it recruits and retains a workforce which has the capacity, perspective, skills, diversity and flexibility to meet the demands on the service. In doing so, managers will need to

Box 1.4 Principal elements of an equality strategy

- Clear commitment to challenge and rejection of discrimination.
- Review established policies and procedures.
- Consultation and involvement of communities in the planning and delivery of services.
- Drafting strategies, objectives, action plans and timescales.
- Implementation of strategy.
- Allocation of responsibility to a senior manager.
- Allocation of necessary resources.
- Monitoring the impact of the strategy.

identify discrimination and inequality, recognise the effects of past discrimination and the exclusion or underrepresentation of different sections of society. Most importantly, however, it needs to value differences and treat people in ways which bring out the best in them.

It could be argued that all the tenets of change management, including a comprehensive strategy for action and long-term commitment, apply universally to the nurse manager in the management of diversity and inequalities and that no special or unusual action is required. For the nurse manager, the principles involved are thus very similar to those used in delivering patient care. Just as a nurse assesses a patient before setting goals, planning interventions, carrying out appropriate actions and evaluating the results, addressing diversity and inequality requires the nurse manager to assess a situation, set goals for staff or groups of patients, develop and implement a plan of action and evaluate the outcome (Box 1.4).

Wider policy agenda

Managers will need to take account of the wider management agendas within their service. The goals of the government's modernisation agenda for the health service are thus very important in this context (Secretary of State for Health 1997). In relation to human resources, the goal is to increase staff numbers and to build capacity and capability in the management of people and organisational change and to improve the working life for staff (DoH 1998, 1999a). In terms of service delivery, the government's strategy for addressing inequalities (DoH 1999b) and its plans for strengthening the role of the nurse in the new NHS (DoH 1999c) provide the backdrop against which nurse managers can develop strategic action. Health improvement programmes are the local strategies for improving health and health care (Donald 1999); all local policies likely to have a direct or indirect effect on health are evaluated in terms of their impact on health inequalities and are formulated in such a way that by favouring the less well off they will, wherever possible, reduce such inequalities. Health authorities are required to play a leadership role to stimulate the development of policies beyond the boundaries of the NHS and to work in partnership with local authorities, the voluntary and business sectors to involve local people in developing and providing services (NHS Executive 1998).

Essential skills in diversity competence

The link between quality management of staff and quality service delivery is now well recognised. Thus, if effective, such strategies should change the profile of the top tier of management to reflect the picture within the wider society and result in more flexible and inclusive professional practices. The inevitable conflict generated by such changes will need to be managed effectively. The development of particular competencies is thus essential if managers are not to be constrained. Three skills which those without previous training will have to develop are values clarification, cultural communication and leadership. These will be briefly discussed below.

Values clarification

Values clarification helps nurse managers to become aware of personal beliefs and principles so that they can examine, select and learn to act on a specific ideology. This process increases self-awareness and self-confidence, helps reaffirm a commitment to goals, improves decision-making skills and guides behavioural changes (Grant & Massey 1999). Awareness of one's own viewpoint and values is as vital to success as the ability to employ capable staff, deal with the finances and with organisational restructuring.

The professional codes of ethics that guide the nurse manager are important in this process. Registered nurses may look to the UKCC *Code of professional conduct* (UKCC 1992) and other UKCC documents for guidelines regarding their values-based actions in relation to patients/clients and staff. Item 7 of this code expects nurses to recognise and respect the uniqueness and dignity of each patient and client and respond to their need for care, irrespective of their ethnic origin, religious beliefs, personal attributes, the nature of their health problem or any other factor.

Grant & Massey (1999) describe seven steps involved in values clarifications as follows.

1. Examining personal, emotional, intellectual and physical responses to experiences and interactions with others.
2. Distinguishing between responses from internal (self) and external (others) sources.
3. Reflecting on internal responses for consistency with personal values.
4. Accepting the need for change in attitude or behaviour for consistency with personal values.
5. Evaluating alternative ways to achieve these changes.
6. Developing behaviour patterns consistent with internal responses and personal values.
7. Developing trust in personal feelings and intuition.

Cultural communication skills

Cultural differences are likely to compound communication (Anderson 1983). Constructive dialogue between people of different cultures is possible only when speakers and listeners understand that the meaning of any communication resides not just in the message but also in the minds of the sender and receiver (McLaren 1999). Even when a speaker and listener come from the same background, they may interpret a message differently according to their personality, their accumulated experience or even their mood of the moment. When they are from different backgrounds, the potential for the message to mean different things is greatly increased.

This underlines the central importance of transcultural communication skills to the NHS, a multicultural microcosm for over 50 years. The extent of cultural diversity will be evident in the differing worldviews, verbal and non-verbal codes of social behaviour, communication styles and expectations of those interacting. Within the health care setting, linguistic differences, differing values and attitudes towards family, work, leisure and different dress and hygiene customs, among other things, will be particularly important. These issues can be highly sensitive and offer a variety of challenges to managers. The pursuit of uniformity has been a long-standing barrier to achieving cultural sensitivity and effective crosscultural communication within the NHS. The task for nurse managers, however, is to place emphasis on bringing together what is best in all the diverse cultures to enhance the quality of staff interaction and patient care.

Effective intercultural communication skills are thus a highly valued asset. McEnrue (1993) describes their characteristics as follows.

- The capacity to accept the relativity of one's own knowledge and perceptions.
- The capacity to be non-judgemental.
- A tolerance for ambiguity.
- The capacity to appreciate and communicate respect for other people's ways, backgrounds, values and beliefs.
- The capacity to demonstrate empathy.
- The capacity to be flexible.
- A willingness to acquire new patterns of behaviour and belief.
- The humility to acknowledge what one does not know.

Leadership

Staff are likely to have a variety of views about how things ought to be done so the manager will be required to take a leadership role. A sound understanding of the concerns of staff is important in creating loyalty and respect. However, as leaders, managers will also have a clear vision of what things should be like in the organisation when diversity is valued, remain confident in their abilities, be able to share this vision with staff and to motivate them to take action to achieve the desired outcomes.

Just as confidence and enthusiasm are contagious, insecurity can be sensed and targeted by some staff. Leaders must be perceptive and use their powers of observation when evaluating the staff's cohesiveness. Early adoption of a leadership style that is effective for both staff and manager provides order and security and supports growth in what can often be a highly stressful atmosphere.

Bethel (1990) summarises that a leader:

- has a mission that matters
- is a big thinker
- has high ethics
- masters change
- is sensitive
- is a risk taker
- is a decisions maker

Diversity and inequality in health and health care

Six Steps to **Effective Management**

- uses power wisely
- communicates effectively
- is courageous
- is a team builder
- is committed.

CONCLUSION

The link between good management of staff and the delivery of quality service is now well recognised. Managing diversity and inequality in the NHS is based on the recognition that there is a need to create change towards an agenda which promotes the values of inclusion and equity and treating people in ways which bring out the best in them. Whereas in the past, the aspects of discrimination and legal obligations were highlighted in equal opportunities initiatives, in recent years organisations are increasingly appreciating that initiatives to address this agenda stand a better chance of success when they are developed from the premise of organisational goals and performance.

Key issues for nurse managers in this context are the skills of values clarification, cultural communication and leadership, the government's plans for modernising the NHS providing a framework for strategic direction.

Discussion questions

The movement in the NHS towards an agenda which promotes the values of inclusion, diversity, and equity and assessment of local and individual needs demands that nurse managers reflect consistently on the following.

- Am I supporting the status quo and conventional norms or aiming for social change?
- Which values imposed by my organisation would I agree with even where they are not accepted by other staff or clients? Which would I dispute?
- Do I recognise and capitalise on the diversity among the staff? How could I improve on this?
- Do I know the health needs of the client group(s) in my care? How can I find out?
- What additional skills do I need?

References

Acheson D (Chair) 1998 Independent Inquiry into Inequalities in Health report. Stationery Office, London

Anderson L R 1983 Management of mixed-cultural work group. Journal of Social Psychology 69:305–319

Audit Commission 1997 Finders, keepers: the management of staff turnover in NHS trusts. Audit Commission, London

Bailey A M 1994 A handicap of negative attitudes and lack of choice: caring for inpatients with disabilities. Professional Nurse September: 786–788

Bartlett C A, Ghoshal S 1989 Managing across boundaries: the transnational solution. Harvard Business School Preview, Boston

Bartz D E, Hillman L, Leher S, Mayhugh G M 1990 A model for managing workforce diversity. Management Education and Development 21(5):321–326

Baxter C, Baxter D 2000 Serious neurological disorders and minority ethnic people: a problem service access needs immediate attention. Public Health Medicine 2(2):76–82

Berry-Lound D J 1993 A carer's guide to eldercare. Host Consultancy, Horsham

Bethel S 1990 Making a difference: 12 qualities that make you a leader. Putnam, New York

Beveridge W 1942 Social insurance and allied services. HMSO, London

Black D, Morris J, Smith C, Townsend P 1980 Inequalities in health: report of a Research Working Group. DHSS, London

Bowler I 1993 They are not the same as us. Midwives' stereotypes of South Asian descent maternity patients. Sociology of Health and Illness 15(2):157–178

Brillhart B, Jay H, Wyers W E 1990 Attitudes towards people with disabilities. Rehabilitation Nursing 15(2):80–82/85

Brown H, Turk V, Stein J 1994 Sexual abuse of adults with learning difficulties. Social Care Research Findings 46. Joseph Rowntree Foundation, York

Calori R 1988 How successful companies manage diverse businesses. Long Range Planning (UK) 3:80–90

Centre for Research in Ethnic Relations 1993 Ethnic minorities in Great Britain: age and gender structure. 1991 Census Statistics. Paper No 2. University of Warwick, Coventry

Cox T H, Blake S 1990 Affirmative action and the issues of expectancies. Journal of Social Issues 46(2):61–67

Davidson M J 1991 Women managers in Britain – issues for the 1990s. Women in Management Review 6(1):5–10

Department of Employment 1988 Employment for the 1990s. HMSO, London

Department of Health 1998 Working together: securing a quality workforce for the NHS. DoH, London

Department of Health 1999a Improving working lives. DoH, London

Department of Health 1999b Reducing inequalities in the NHS: an action report. Stationery Office, London

Department of Health 1999c Making a difference: strengthening the nursing, midwifery and health visiting contribution to health and healthcare. DoH, London

Donald A 1999 Becoming the future: changing clinical behaviour. In: Rawaf S (ed) Health improvement programmes: the millennium approach to health and healthcare. Royal Society of Medicine, London

Donaldson L 1993 The recession: a barrier to equal opportunities? Equal Opportunities Review 50:1–16

Ellison R 1994 British labour force projections: 1994 to 2006. Employment Gazette April:111–122

Equal Opportunities Review 1997 Equality for lesbians and gay men in the workplace. Journal of Management 16(1):107–118

Galagan P A 1991 Tapping the power of a diverse workforce. Training and Development Journal 45(3):38–44

Gold M, Campbell A 1987 Managing diversity: strategy and control in diversified British companies. Long Range Planning 20(5):42–52

Grant A B, Massey V H 1999 Nursing leadership, management and research. Springhouse, Pennsylvania

Hall D, Parker V A 1993 The role of workplace flexibility in managing diversity. Organisational Dynamics 22(1):4–18

Hammond T R, Kleiner B H 1992 Managing multicultural work environments. Equal Opportunities International 11(2):6–9

Honey S, Meager N, Williams M 1993 Employers' attitudes towards people with disabilities. BEPC, Dorset

Jameson D, O'Mara J 1991 Managing workforce 2000: work gaining the diversity advantage. Jossey-Bass, San Francisco

Kandola R, Fullerton J 1998 Diversity in action. Institute of Personnel Development, London

Kennedy J, Everest A 1991 Putting diversity into context. Personnel Journal September:50–54

Labour Force Survey 1997 Labour Force Survey quarterly bulletin, December 22. Office of National Statistics, London

Lalonde M 1974 A new perspective in the health of Canadians. Office of the Canadian Minister of National Health and Welfare, Ottawa

Larbie J 1984 Black women and maternity services: training in health and race. National Extension College, Cambridge

Lynch F R 1994 Workforce diversity: PC's final frontier? National Review 46(3):32

McEnrue M P 1993 Managing diversity: Los Angeles before and after the riots. Organisational Dynamics 21(3):18–29

McLaren C M 1999 Interpreting cultural differences: the challenge of intercultural communication. Peter Francis Publishers, Norwich

McNaught A 1985 Race and health in the United Kingdom. Occasional Paper No 2. Health Education Council, London

New Ways to Work 1993 Change at the top: working flexibly at senior and managerial levels in organisations. New Ways to Work, London

NHS Executive 1998 Planning for better health and better healthcare. National Health Service Circular 1998/167. NHSE, Leeds

Paine L S 1994 Managing for organisational integrity. Harvard Business Review 72(2):106–117

Payne J 1991 Women, training and skills shortage. PSI, London

Phillips N 1992 Managing international teams. Pitman Publishing, London

Platzer H 1993 Nursing care of gay and lesbian patients. Nursing Standard 7(17):34–37

Ross R, Schneider R 1992 From diversity to equality: a business case for equal opportunities. Pitman Publishing, London

Secretary of State for Health 1997 The new NHS: modern, dependable. Stationery Office, London

Syrett M, Lammiman J 1994 Developing the peripheral worker. Personnel Management July: 28–31

Thomas R R 1991 Beyond race and gender: unleashing the power of your total workforce by managing diversity. AMOCAM, New York

Townsend P, Whitehead M, Davidson N 1992 Introduction to inequalities in health. In: Townsend P, Whitehead M, Davidson N (eds) Inequalities in health: the Black Report and the Health Divide, 2nd edn. Penguin, London

Trompena F 1993 Riding the waves of culture: understanding cultural diversity in business. Economist Books, London

Turk V, Brown H 1992 Sexual abuse and adults with learning disabilities. Mental Handicap 20(2):56–58

United Kingdom Central Council 1992 Code of professional conduct for nurses, midwives and health visitors. UKCC, London

Whitehead M 1995 Tackling inequalities: a review of policy initiatives. In: Benzeval M, Judge K, Whitehead M (eds) Tackling inequalities in health: an agenda for action. King's Fund, London

Whitehead M 1997 Life and death over the millennium. In: Drever F, Whitehead M (eds) Health inequalities: decennial supplement. DS Series No. 15. Stationery Office, London

World Health Organization 1978 Primary health care report of the International Conference on Primary Health Care, Alma-Ata, 6–12 September 1978. WHO, Geneva

World Health Organization 1984 Report of the Working Group on Concepts and Principles of Health Promotion. WHO, Copenhagen

World Health Organization 1985a Social justice and equity in health: a report from the Programme on Social Equity and Health. WHO meeting, Leeds, 22–27 July

World Health Organization 1985b Targets for health for all. WHO, Copenhagen

Diversity and inequality in health and health care

Application **1:1**

Sam Ayer

Vulnerability and abuse

WHO ARE VULNERABLE ADULTS?

Within a diverse population, there are some individuals who can be described as vulnerable. Vulnerability often refers to an individual's propensity to experience harm, a vulnerable person being regarded as 'capable of being physically or emotionally wounded or injured; open to successful attack; capable of being persuaded or tempted' (*Chambers English dictionary* 1990). Vulnerable people are not a homogeneous group and arriving at a definition of vulnerability which is neither under- nor overinclusive presents some difficulties.

However, vulnerability is in practice a combination of the characteristics of the people concerned and the risks to which they are exposed by their circumstances. For some people their vulnerability is the result of physical disability where the people concerned cannot protect themselves from unwanted restraint. For others, a deterioration of memory or alertness prevents them from asking for the services which would enable them to live as independent a life as possible. Others may be in an abusive relationship with their carers or other persons and may require care as well as protection and support.

The Lord Chancellor's Department consultation paper defines a vulnerable adult as a person who:

> ...is or may be in need of community care services by reason of mental or other disability, age or illness and who is or may be unable to take care of himself or herself or unable to protect himself or herself against significant harm or exploitation. (Law Commission 1997)

In this paper 'adult' refers to a person aged 18 and over. People with learning disabilities, people with mental health problems as well as older people and people with physical disability or impairment will be included within this definition, particularly when their situation is complicated by additional factors such as physical frailty or chronic illness, sensory impairment, challenging behaviour, drug or alcohol problems, social or emotional problems, poverty or homelessness.

This chapter looks at the forms such abuse of vulnerable adults can take and the responsibility of nurses in protecting the interests of

Diversity and inequality in health care

vulnerable patients and sets out the implications for nursing management.

THE ABUSE OF VULNERABLE ADULTS

The abuse of a vulnerable adult may consist of a single act or repeated acts over time. It may occur as a result of a failure to undertake action or appropriate care tasks. It may be physical, psychological or an act of neglect or occur where a vulnerable person is persuaded to enter into a financial or sexual transaction to which they have not or cannot consent.

Abuse can occur in any relationship and may result in significant harm to or exploitation of the individual. In everyday nursing situations nurses encounter two groups who are particularly vulnerable. People with learning disabilities and with mental health problems are at risk of abuse because of their vulnerability. Such abuse can take many forms.

- *Physical abuse* – this includes hitting, slapping, pushing, kicking, misuse of medication, restraint or inappropriate sanctions.
- *Sexual abuse* – this includes rape and sexual assault or sexual acts to which the vulnerable person has not or could not consent and/or to which they are pressured into consenting.
- *Psychological abuse* – this includes emotional abuse, threats of harm or abandonment, deprivation of contact, humiliation, blaming, controlling, intimidation, coercion, verbal or racial abuse, isolation or withdrawal from services or support networks.
- *Financial or material abuse* – this includes theft, fraud, exploitation, pressure in connection with wills, property or inheritance or financial transactions or the misuse or misappropriation of property, possessions or benefits.
- *Neglect and acts of omission* – this includes ignoring medical or physical care needs or failure to provide access to appropriate health, nursing and social care or educational services, the withholding of the necessities of life, such as medication, adequate nutrition and heating (DoH 1999, McCreadie 1994, Williams 1994).

NURSING MANAGEMENT OF VULNERABLE PEOPLE WITH LEARNING DISABILITIES AND PEOPLE WITH MENTAL HEALTH PROBLEMS

The closure of institutions and the integration of people with learning disabilities and people with mental health problems into the community has meant that work with these client groups takes place in a variety of settings including ordinary family settings, residential

Vulnerability and abuse

and inpatient setting run by voluntary and private organisations, day-care settings run by health trusts and social services department. Nursing staff work in these settings together with other non-nursing staff and carers, many of whom have not undergone any recognised or formalised course of training.

Nurse managers have overall duties as registered nurses to maintain public trust and confidence in their ability to provide safe and effective care for their clients. Professional accountability is fundamentally concerned with weighing up the interests of the client and using professional judgement and skills to make decisions and to account for such decisions. Nurse managers are accountable for ensuring that their knowledge and skills are up to date.

Accountability is an integral part of professional practice. In the course of professional practice nurse managers will have to make judgements in a wide variety of circumstances with regards to their professional responsibilities in order to safeguard and promote the best interests of individual clients and serve the interests of society.

Consent

Valid consent consists of three elements: it is given by a competent person who may be lawfully appointed on behalf of the client, it is given voluntarily and it is informed (UKCC 1998). Nurse managers have three overriding professional responsibilities with regard to obtaining consent.

- They must act in the best interests of the client and obtain consent before they give any treatment or care.
- They must ensure that the process of establishing consent is rigorous and transparent and demonstrates a clear level of professional accountability.
- All discussions and decisions relating to consent must be recorded accurately.

Working in a collaborative and cooperative manner

In the exercise of professional accountability the manager must work in a collaborative and cooperative manner with health care professionals and others involved in providing care and recognise and respect their particular contributions within the interprofessional and multidisciplinary care team.

The *Code of professional conduct* requires the nurse manager to 'report to an appropriate person or authority any circumstances in which safe and appropriate care for the clients cannot be provided' (UKCC 1992).

Promoting and safeguarding the clients' interests

Nurse managers should endeavour to promote and safeguard the clients' interests. They should be clear about their role in advocating for clients and should establish whether clients have particular needs which are not being addressed. This will include considering clients' physical, emotional, cultural and religious beliefs and recognising issues of racial discrimination and disadvantage. Identifying these needs requires the ability to listen to clients and respond in the most appropriate way. For example, the manager may wish to support the client in seeking an independent advocate.

Professional practice is based upon the manager developing a therapeutic relationship with clients. Such a relationship should not only promote client independence and autonomy but also promote and safeguard the clients' rights to choose and empower them to be involved in decision making.

CONCLUSION

As care moves away from hospital and into a range of alternative and diverse settings, preventing the abuse of vulnerable adults with mental health problems and/or learning disabilities becomes a major professional and ethical issue for the nurse manager. As a recent Department of Health consultation document points out:

> A key element and the starting point for successfully dealing with concerns and allegations of the abuse of vulnerable adults must be that agencies have *an organisational environment and framework within which all concerned feel able to come forward without fear of ridicule, victimisation or other negative consequence.* Without this the risk of abuse going unnoticed, unreported and thus continuing will remain. (emphasis in original, DoH 1999, p 27)

Discussion questions

In your role as a nurse manager, reflect on the following.
- What forms of adult abuse might exist in your workplace?
- What policies exist to ensure that staff are able to expose bad practice?
- What training regime exists in your organisation to ensure recognition of the incidence of bad practice, ill treatment and other forms of abuse?
- Is there a policy of whistle blowing in your organisation?
- What are the pros and cons of developing a standard policy for whistle blowing applicable in the multidisciplinary and interprofessional care settings?

Vulnerability and abuse

References

Chambers English Dictionary 1990 Chambers, Edinburgh

Department of Health 1999 No secrets: the protection of vulnerable adults. DoH, London

Law Commission 1997 Who decides? Making decisions on behalf of mentally incapacitated adults. Stationery Office, London

McCreadie C 1994 The nature of abuse. In: Eastman M (ed) Old age abuse: a new perspective. Chapman and Hall, London

UKCC 1992 Code of professional conduct. UKCC, London

UKCC 1998 Guidelines for mental health and learning disabilities nursing. UKCC, London

Williams C 1994 Invisible victims. Jessica Kingsley, London

Diversity and inequality in health care

Application **1.2**

Jo Alleyne, Mansour Jumaa

Equal opportunities agreements and monitoring in NHS Trusts

INTRODUCTION

The government is committed to the development of a more strategic, service-wide approach to the management of human resources in the NHS and in particular to the development of the nursing, midwifery and health-visiting workforce. A recent review of workforce planning in England has reported that the government's commitments to the expansion of the numbers of health professionals must also include reforms; in the way that people work, the way they are trained and how they are educated (DoH 2000).

If we are to achieve the aim of developing a workforce which recognises the talents of its staff, then equal opportunities (EO) should be a mainstreamed activity, reflected throughout the strategies, structures, systems, skills, styles and staff within the health service. It should be demonstrated through the core values of each health service organisation and operationalised and recognised as 'the way we do things around here'.

In October 1997, Industrial Relations Services Research was commissioned by the NHS Equal Opportunities Unit to carry out a survey of equal opportunities agreements and monitoring in the NHS trusts in England (NHS Equal Opportunities Unit 1998). The findings of the survey are presented below.

SURVEY PROFILE

A total of 420 out of 425 trusts responded, a 98.9% response rate, broken down as follows:

- 46% acute trusts
- 27% community trusts
- 8% mental health trusts
- 8% combined or integrated trusts

- 9% ambulance trusts
- 2% learning disabilities trusts.

EQUAL OPPORTUNITIES STRUCTURE WITHIN THE TRUSTS

- The main EO responsibility at senior management level was found in the human resources department: 82% of trusts' responsibility lay with the HR/personnel director.
- Only 10 (2%) of trusts had a specialist post dedicated to EO in employment.
- The vast majority of trusts do have a member of staff whose overall responsibilities include EO in employment.
- Just under three-quarters of trusts (310) reported that they have a joint staff/management forum to progress EO in employment issues.

EQUAL OPPORTUNITIES AGREEMENTS

The vast majority of trusts – 412 (98%) – have a general policy statement which covers EO in employment. Of trusts with a general EO policy:

- 96% have a policy on maternity pay and leave
- >90% specifically covered ethnic minority, disabled and female employees
- 81% covered employees of different faiths
- 80% have policies on recruitment and selection, carer leave, adoption leave, paternity leave and harassment by other staff
- 70% have policies on job sharing
- smaller proportions have policies on harassment by patients (59%), retainer schemes (38%), childcare and other special leave (38%), older employees (67%) HIV/AIDS (51%), phased return to work after illness (31%), bullying at work (23%).

An analysis by type of trust shows that:

- a smaller proportion of ambulance trusts have certain policies, particularly those covering specified types of leave, than trusts as a whole
- a slightly higher proportion of acute trusts and integrated trusts have policies on most of the specified subject areas, compared with trusts as a whole
- a slightly higher proportion of community trusts have policies on the different types of leave (e.g. adoption and special leave) than trusts as a whole
- a smaller proportion of learning disabilities trusts have policies in a number of areas (including harassment by staff and harassment

by patients, job sharing and retainer schemes), compared with trusts as a whole. However, there are only 10 trusts in the survey in this category.

MONITORING OF RECRUITMENT PROCESS

Over 90% of trusts collect information on job applicants by gender, ethnic origin and disability, the proportions being distributed as follows:

- 92% collect monitoring information on the ethnic origin of those appointed
- 90% collect data on appointments by gender
- 88% collect data on disabled people.

WORKFORCE PROFILE MONITORING

The majority of trusts collected monitoring data on the total workforce by gender, ethnic origin, disability and whether employed part time or full time.

Only a minority of trusts collected monitoring data on promotion, redundancies, dismissals or training.

Discussion questions

Managers attempting to take policy initiatives forward will find it useful to reflect on the following.

- Is there anything significant about these findings and why?
- How would you rate your organisation's performance on equal opportunities?
- How familiar are you with your own trust's equal opportunities policy?
- How might things have changed in your organisation since this survey was carried out?
- What proportion of nurses in your organisation are from the various minority groups?
- Is diversity reflected across all nursing disciplines in your organisation?
- Which equality issue is a priority for your organisation?

References

Department of Health 2000 A health service of all the talents: developing the NHS workforce. Consultation Document on the Review of Workforce Planning. DoH, London

NHS Equal Opportunities Unit 1998 Equal opportunities and monitoring in NHS trusts. NHSE, Leeds

Equal opportunities agreements and monitoring in NHS Trusts

Application 1:3

John James, Carol Baxter

The Organisational Effectiveness Perspective in recruitment and selection: reflecting on a model from the private sector

INTRODUCTION

An expansion in numbers, enhancing competence and promoting values of inclusion and equity amongst its workforce are major themes within the current government strategy for modernising the NHS. In particular, to meet nursing shortfalls, high-profile attention is currently being given to recruiting staff from all sections of society, with international recruitment being actively pursued. A recent intensification of the recruitment campaign will undoubtedly bring to the fore issues in relation to how hiring decisions are made.

Based on experiences in private sector organisations in the USA, Powell (1998) puts forward the Organisational Effectiveness Perspective (OEP) as a framework for managers in the human resource field to make hiring decisions. This chapter discusses the OEP and encourages the reader to reflect on its usefulness in the context of the NHS.

THE ORGANISATIONAL EFFECTIVENESS PERSPECTIVE

The OEP is based on two distinct paradigms: the organisational cohesiveness and organisational diversity models. The former promotes a selection strategy where hiring decisions are based on employees who reflect and reinforce the existing core values and culture of the organisation – referred to as 'reinforcing fit'. The organisational diversity model, on the other hand, favours hiring decisions which actively seek out new employees to increase diversity, thus extending the range of the organisation's strengths – referred to as 'extending fit'.

These two models appear to present competing paradigms for how to achieve organisational success: their strengths and weaknesses are outlined in Table 1.3.1.

The OEP is designed to ensure that the organisation recruits new employees who will help it to do what it already does well and to recruit new employees to do things that it has never done before.

This perspective draws on both the cohesiveness and diversity models. Powell (1998) asserts that the simultaneous pursuit of

Table 1.3.1 Cohesiveness and diversity models (adapted from Powell 1998)

Model	Advantages	Disadvantages
Organisational cohesiveness	• Enhances the organisation's culture. • Important when there is a rapid pace of change and in situations such as mergers.	• A vague definition of fit may result in selection decisions which favour the dominant demographic group. • Job candidates who are astute at impression management can sense what the interviewers are looking for. • Recruiters favour job candidates who they see as similar to themselves. • Preserves the organisation's historical demographics. • Slow in responding to the need for environmental change.
Organisational diversity	• More sensitivity to a variety of markets. • Quicker in responding to changes. • More creative solutions to problems. • Broadens organisational perspective and culture.	• Erodes organisational cohesiveness. • Often exhibits dysfunctional team processes. • Minorities subjected to stereotypes and performance pressures.

Six Steps to **Effective Management**

reinforcing and extending fit can help the organisation respond to different types of concerns, thus enhancing overall organisational effectiveness (see Table 1.3.2). He suggests that when hiring staff, managers adhere to a number of important principles in determining when it is appropriate to pursue either reinforcing or extending philosophy and that this can be done by addressing the following three questions.

- Fit on what personal attributes?
- Fit for employees in which jobs?
- Fit in what situations?

Table 1.3.2 The simultaneous pursuit of reinforcing and extending fit (adapted from Powell 1998)

Question	Search for reinforcing fit	Search for extending fit
Fit on what personal attributes?	● On values that are pivotal to the organisation's culture ● On general types of knowledge, skills and abilities (**KSAs**)	● On specific types of KSAs that are needed to perform different types of jobs ● On specific types of KSAs that are needed to solve different types of problems ● On specific types of KSAs which are needed to take advantage of different types of opportunities
Fit for employees in which jobs?	● For employees at lower levels who neither hold nor are expected to hold jobs with decision-making responsibilities	● For employees at lower levels who either hold or are expected to hold jobs with decision-making responsibilities ● For employees at higher levels who hold jobs with decision-making responsibilities
Fit in what situations?	● When the organisation is at an early stage in its lifecycle ● When the industry is in a state of equilibrium and is likely to remain so ● When the department or organisation has a low degree of contact with consumers ● When the department or organistion serves similar customers	● When the organisation is at a later stage of its lifecycle ● When the industry is subject to periods of revolutionary change at short notice ● When the department or organisation has a high degree of contact with customers ● When the department or organisation serves diverse customers

BASIC PRINCIPLES

The extract below is Powell's discussion of the basic principles which managers are advised to consider in determining when the pursuit of each type of fit is best for the organisation. (Reproduced from Powell G N 1998 Reinforcing and extending today's organisations: the simultaneous pursuit of person–organisation fit and diversity. Organisational Dynamics 26(3):50-61 with permission from Elsevier Science.)

Search for reinforcing fit on pivotal values but do not bother searching for reinforcing or extending fit on peripheral values

Not all values that may be represented in an organisation's culture are critical to its success. Scheirn (1988) distinguished between pivotal values, which are essential to the organisation's success, and peripheral values, which have become associated with the organisation's culture for historical reasons rather than for their contribution to its success. For example, the pivotal values for business schools include expectations that staff members will keep abreast with developments through their consulting. In some business schools, it is also expected that staff will wear 'normal business attire' during the conduct of their responsibilities. The latter expectation is not critical to the success of the business school and thus represents a peripheral value. Similarly, norms regarding work attire have been relaxed in many organisations in recent years. Even IBM, once known for having one of the strictest dress codes of any large organisation, no longer stresses adherence to rigid standards of dress as a pivotal value.

Searching for reinforcing fit on pivotal values is a good way for an organisation to preserve the key elements of its culture. In fact, adherence to similar consideration of values such as mutual respect, openness, participation and consideration of alternative points of view facilitates a multicultural approach to diversity. On the other hand, searching for either reinforcing or extending fit on peripheral values seems unnecessary. Employees need to be allowed to express themselves as they wish, as long as they exhibit the pivotal values that support the organisation's mission.

Search for reinforcing fit on general KSAs but search for extending fit on specific KSAs that are needed to perform different types of jobs and respond to different types of problems and opportunities

A study of college recruiters identified that they generally looked for such traits as good communication skills, cognitive ability, cooperative attitude, work ethic and self-confidence. These are, however, generally desirable rather than specific to the needs of any one organisation. Thus searching for reinforcing fit on that basis seems appropriate. However, a variety of specific KSAs are necessary for specific work to be done well and it is not necessary for any employee to possess all of them. To state an obvious example, an airline should have some employees with the KSAs needed to fly planes and others with KSAs needed to provide information about flight schedules and sell tickets to customers. But it is not necessary for pilots to be able to serve as ticketing agents or vice versa. Although the trend in high involvement organisations is to encourage job rotation and sharing of KSAs, few organisations will ever apply job rotation to all jobs.

Variety in personal characteristics such as functional area and work experience can bring to the table different types of KSAs that are needed to enhance the organisation's performance capabilities. When the problem to be solved involves several functions, diversity in the kinds of expertise and experience that employees possess can help the organisation arrive at innovative solutions. The same kind of diversity can also enhance the organisation's readiness to exploit new market opportunities as they arise. Thus it is appropriate to search for extending fit for the organisation as a whole so that the employees collectively possess the various types of jobs, solve different types of problems and take advantage of different types of opportunities.

Search for reinforcing fit for employees at lower levels who neither hold nor are expected to hold jobs with decision-making responsibilities, but search for extending fit for employees who currently hold (or are expected to hold) jobs with decision-making responsibilities

The more important the problem to be solved or decision to be made, the greater the benefits of diversity. Thus, the search for extending fit seems most useful for the top management team and for others who determine the organisation's mission and strategy. Also, if the organisation is centralised with most key decisions made at the top, the greatest benefits of diversity may be achieved at the top.

When lower level employees are primarily responsible for implementing decisions made by others, searching for reinforcing fit facilitates their acting in a consistent manner to implement these decisions. However, if responsibilities for decisions are delegated to lower level employees, then the search for extending fit becomes useful at lower levels as well. In addition, when lower level employees are seen as having a reasonable chance of holding positions with greater decision-making responsibilities in the future, the search for extending fit is appropriate. This will contribute to the development of a pool of employees who will be ready to move into such positions when the opportunity arises.

Diversity and inequality in health care

Search for reinforcing fit in early stages of the organisation's lifecycle, but search for extending fit in later stages of the lifecycle

Having a strong culture may not be equally desirable for organisations at all times. An extensive study of 28 firms, for example, shows that a strong organisational culture is associated with better performance over the short run. However, over the long run, particularly when an organisation's environment changes rapidly, a strong culture compromises the firm's ability to adapt effectively.

Consistency in employees' personalities and values, achieved by searching for high reinforcing fit, helps organisations to be successful early in their history because it creates the cohesiveness and sense of cooperation required for success; as organisations sustain their success over time, such consistency can result in inflexibility and inability to change when necessary. In other words, a company's core capabilities (including its knowledge, skills, systems, processes and values) can become core rigidities unless adapted to changing conditions over time.

Sears, for example, developed a strong culture based on its successes through the 1960s that kept later Chief Executive Officers from making radical changes that were needed to respond to shifting consumer preferences. On the other hand, Wal-Mart, which was less restrained by its past, prospered during the same time period. Thus, searching for reinforcing fit may be more useful to organisations at early stages in their lifecycles when they are struggling to achieve initial success; extending fit may be more useful at later stages as a response to changing conditions in the marketplace.

Search for reinforcing fit when the organisation is in an industry that is expected to remain in a state of equilibrium, but search for extending fit when the organisation is in an industry that is subject to periods of revolutionary change at short notice

Industries vary in the rates at which they exhibit change, whether the change is driven by innovative technologies that transform the production process (for example, new ways of making steel) or consumer demands that call for innovative products or services (e.g. digital television reception via satellite). Organisations characterised by reinforcing fit will be more successful when only gradual change is needed to keep up with the rest of the industry. When the industry is rapidly changing, organisations characterised by extending fit will be better able to anticipate these changes and to stay ahead of competitors.

However, many industries change at an uneven rate. They go through long periods of equilibrium that call only for incremental changes, then enter periods of upheaval that call for revolutionary changes. Connie Gersick (1991) observed that the difference between the incremental changes of equilibrium periods and revolutionary

The Organisational Effectiveness Perspective in recruitment and selection changes is like the difference between changing the game of basketball by raising the hoops, compared with removing the hoops. The first kind of change leaves the basic structure of the game intact while calling for adjustments in how the game is played. The second type of change alters the essential nature of the game and calls for completely different rules.

To be ready to play fundamentally different games at short notice, organisations need to keep themselves from being overly committed to one particular strategy. Searching for extending fit, particularly in the top management team, will help to keep an organisation ready to respond to revolutionary periods of change when they arise, even if the industry is in a state of equilibrium. However, searching for reinforcing fit will help keep an organisation successful when periods of revolutionary change seem unlikely.

Search for reinforcing fit when the department or organisation has a low degree of contact with customers and serves similar customers, but search for extending fit when the department or organisation has a high degree of contact with customers and serves diverse communities or departments

Organisations differ in their degree of contact with customers, as do departments or work units within a company. In product organisations, no matter whether the product is soup or sailboats, production is carried out with an awareness of customers' needs, but production employees typically do not interact with customers. In these same companies, however, employees in the marketing and sales departments are likely to have contact with customers. Conversely, in service organisations, no matter whether the service is health care or financial advice, employees in a variety of departments have the opportunity to interact with customers.

In addition, the potential customers for any product may belong to diverse groups with diverse needs for products and services or primarily to one group with narrowly defined needs. For example, the average age of Cadillac buyers is now over 60 with few people under 40 saying that they would even consider buying the car. This makes the base of potential Cadillac customers especially homogeneous compared with the potential customers for many other automobiles. When potential customers are concentrated in one group, employees who possess reinforcing fit are believed to know how to respond best to the narrow interests of the particular customer base. When potential customers are widely distributed across diverse groups, however, employees who possess extending fit may better understand the needs of such customers.

Implications for organisations

The implications of the organisational effectiveness perspective are clear: managers should not declare themselves for or against either *reinforcing* or *extending fit.* The single-minded pursuit of either type of fit in hiring new employees is too simplistic. Statements like 'We need to hire new employees who fit our existing organisational culture to compete successfully' or 'We need to hire new employees who increase the diversity of our workforce to compete successfully' are insufficient guidelines by themselves. Instead, managers should consider the three basic questions about fit posed above. Answering the three basic questions posed above will help organisations diagnose their needs for either reinforcing fit or extending fit based on different types of personal attributes (pivotal or peripheral values, general or specific types of knowledge, skills and abilities), different types of jobs (with decision-making responsibilities or not at different levels), and different types of situations (organisational, lifecycle stage, likelihood of revolutionary change in the industry, extent of customer contact, extent of diversity in potential customers).

In implementing their selection strategies organisations need to be sure that they are hiring people with the right characteristics to function well in their particular environment, not members of particular demographic groups whom they assume will possess the right characteristics. They need to take precautions that selecting officials' biases do not lead to decisions which consciously or unconsciously discriminate against any demographic group. Such biases are most likely to prevail when decision-makers are guided by only vague notions of fit. Organisations can avoid this by identifying their pivotal values as precisely as possible and then specifying ways to assess these values in job candidates through the use of personality measures or lines of questioning in interviews.

Organisations also need to caution selecting officials against assuming that applicants who are similar to themselves will make the best employees or applicants with similar demographic characteristics will exhibit similar personal traits. Taking these precautions will enable organisations to hire new employees who possess good levels of both reinforcing fit and extending fit without sacrificing demographic diversity.

Discussion questions

- Private sector organisations in the USA have a longer track record in these issues than the NHS. Are there any advantages in modelling service delivery on this retail concept?
- Consider the above question in relation to your own enterprise and think whether it provides a direct service to users or carers or whether your customers are primarily internal.
- Make notes on the following suggestion: in terms of its current situation, the NHS is required to prioritise its search for extending fit.
- Reflect on the above question in relation to the recruitment and selection of ethnic minorities in the NHS.

The Organisational Effectiveness Perspective in recruitment and selection

Six Steps to **Effective Management**

References

Gersick C J C 1991 Revolutionary change theories: a multilevel exploration of the punctuated equilibrium paradigm. Academy of Management Review 16:10–36

Powell G N 1998 Reinforcing and extending today's organisations: the simultaneous pursuit of person–organisation fit and diversity. Organisational Dynamics 26(3):50–61

Scheirn E H 1988 Organisational socialisation and the profession of management. Sloane Management Review 30(1):53–65

Diversity and inequality in health care

Chapter **Two**

Antiracism, multiculturalism and the third way

Irena Papadopoulos

- ● Introduction
- ● The multicultural explanation
- ● The antiracist explanation
- ● A new unified approach: the third way
- ● Conclusion

OVERVIEW

This chapter considers the two main theoretical perspectives which relate to the health of people from minority ethnic groups. It provides the arguments for and against multiculturalism and antiracism and then moves on to examine the emerging alternative way in ethnic health developments. It is becoming evident that in Britain today, ethnic health is being located within the broader framework of inequalities in health, social exclusion and an emphasis on citizenship rights and responsibilities. The chapter concludes that it is too early to make any judgement as to whether this 'third way' will be more successful than previous attempts.

INTRODUCTION

Kelleher (1996) maintains that in Britain today there are two positions from which the analysis around patterns of ethnic health and health variations is conducted: the multiculturalist position and the antiracist position. The multiculturalist position, whilst not denying the existence of racism, attempts to emphasise both the existence and the validity of different cultural traditions amongst ethnic groups. From this perspective, it is argued that through the promotion of tolerance and understanding of different cultural traditions, appropriate, relevant and culturally sensitive health care will be provided and inevitably this will result in the improvement of health for all ethnic groups and that of the majority population. Supporters of the antiracists, on the other hand, believe that attention to culture acts as a diversion from racism, rather than promoting understanding of cultural diversity. Thus, they argue, health inequalities can only be addressed if more political emphasis is placed on the forces that structure social relationships and determine access to power in society.

It is apparent that there exist ideological differences between the two positions. It also appears that the differences in the two positions may have been exacerbated by the problems surrounding the lack of clarity in the terms used by researchers and academics as they try to expand their knowledge and understanding around the health and illness of people from different minority ethnic groups. This view is supported by, amongst others, Bulmer (1986), McNaught (1987), Crowley & Simmons (1992) and Anthias & Yuval-Davis (1992) who have suggested that the terms associated with minority ethnic groups such as 'culture', 'race' and 'ethnicity' are among the most elusive to define. Sheldon & Parker (1992) have identified a lack of consistency in terminology regarding ethnicity. In addition, McKenzie & Crowcroft (1994) have argued against using ethnicity as a variable in health research, pointing out that this is most problematic in relation to second- and third-generation people who have had considerable contact with the British culture, having been born and educated in Britain.

During the 1980s and early 1990s the ability of health professions to deliver adequate and appropriate health care to Britain's multiracial, multicultural population was questioned (Audit Commission 1992, King's Fund 1990). Torkington (1984) stated that people from minority ethnic groups were at best received with indifference by health professionals but many were exposed to neglect and hostility to their culture. McNaught (1987) and Francis et al (1989) found that in some cases, problems are trivialised and their seriousness not acknowledged whilst in other cases misdiagnosis occurs. The recently published report of the independent Inquiry into Inequalities in Health (Acheson 1998) makes it patently clear that there is a need to train health workers in 'cultural competence'. The report also recommends that further developments of services which are sensitive to the needs of minority ethnic people and which promote greater awareness of their health risks should be implemented.

THE MULTICULTURAL EXPLANATION

According to the multicultural approach, the existing unsatisfactory position in relation to health problems associated with people from minority ethnic groups is due to lack of knowledge and understanding of the various cultural traditions of ethnic groups. But what do we mean by culture and ethnicity? How does one achieve cultural understanding and competence and is the remedy as simple as it sounds?

Culture, according to Tylor (1871), is a complex whole which includes knowledge, belief, art, morals, law, custom and any other capabilities and habits acquired by a person as a member of society. Kessing's (1981) definition stresses the ideational aspect of culture; that is, cultures comprise systems of shared ideas, concepts, rules and meanings that underlie and are expressed in the ways in which humans live. Leininger (1991) also defines culture in similar ways:

> Culture refers to the learned, shared, and transmitted values, beliefs, norms, and lifeways of a particular group that guides their thinking, decisions, and actions in patterned ways. (p 47)

It can thus be argued that culture is a set of guidelines (both explicit and implicit) which individuals inherit as members of a particular society and which tells them how to view the world, how to experience it emotionally and how to behave in it, in relation to other people, to supernatural forces or gods and to the natural environment. It also provides individuals with a way of transmitting these guidelines to the next generation by the use of symbols, language, arts and rituals. To some extent, culture can be seen as an inherited 'lens', through which individuals perceive and understand the world that they inhabit and learn how to live within it (Helman 1990). Growing up within any society is a form of enculturation whereby the individual slowly acquires the cultural lens of

Antiracism, multiculturalism and the third way

that society. Without such a shared perception of the world, both the cohesion and the continuity of any human group would be impossible.

Pfeffer & Moynihan (1996) have suggested that culture and ethnicity are both woolly categories and that they seem to be used interchangeably. Fernando (1991) also believes that ethnicity is a term that lacks precision and suggests that it alludes to the definition of both cultural and racial groups. The overriding feature of an ethnic group is the sense of belonging which individuals may have. This feeling may also be promoted by the way society at large perceives people. If certain persons are seen as belonging together for cultural or racial reasons and are treated as such, a sense of being part of the group may develop. Thus cultural similarity, real or imagined, may engender or even determine someone's ethnicity. Fernando goes on to say that the concept of ethnicity has replaced to some degree both race and culture as a basis for defining groups of people in multicultural, multiracial societies.

Kavanagh & Kennedy (1992) claim that we are all a product of our culture(s). Cultural background therefore has an important influence on many aspects of our lives including, among others, our beliefs, behaviours and attitudes to illness, pain and other forms of misfortunes, all of which may have important implications for health and health care. Dobson (1991) believes that our cultural upbringing can also make us ethnocentric to some degree; we see what our culture permits us to see and we find it difficult to imagine life any other way. However, anthropologists such as Leach (1982) have pointed out that virtually all societies have more than one culture within their borders. Many of these groups will undergo some degree of acculturation, whereby they incorporate some of the cultural attributes of the larger society.

Spector (1991) argues that it is mandatory for health professionals to be able to identify, accept and appreciate the cultural differences of their clients. She goes on to say that health professionals are socialised into the culture of their professions. They are taught a set of beliefs, practices, habits, norms and rituals all of which differ in varying degrees from those of the individual. As they become more knowledgeable, they usually move farther and farther from their past belief systems and farther from the population at large in terms of its understanding and beliefs regarding health and illness. It is not uncommon to hear a patient saying, 'I have no idea what the doctor said'! When people of one belief system about health and illness encounter people with a different belief system, there occurs what is commonly referred to as a 'breakdown in communications'.

Leininger (1978, 1991, 1995), Spector (1991) and Dobson (1991) have argued that knowledge of cultural values is a critical element for nurses if they are to provide appropriate, sensitive and reliable nursing care.

Smaje (1995) also supports the use of culture to study health; however, he warns that culture should not be used as a 'checklist' but as an active social process linked to broader socio-economic patterns. He refers to a number of studies from the developing North American literature which have begun to demonstrate the culturally determined nature of the expression of illness, the resources mobilised to address it and the role of community and religious processes in promoting health (Anderson et al 1989, Kleinman 1987, LaVeist 1993, Levin 1994a, b). In Britain, there have been fewer studies of this kind (Currer 1986, Donovan 1986, Fenton 1985). Smaje suggests that this may reflect the successful campaign by the antiracists to invoke inhibitions about the notion of culture in any researcher interested in this field.

Helman (1990) has argued that the concept of culture has sometimes been misunderstood or even misused. For example, cultures have never been homogeneous and therefore one should always avoid using generalisations in explaining people's beliefs and behaviours. One should therefore differentiate between the rules of a culture which govern how one should think and behave and how people actually behave in real life. Generalisations can also be dangerous for they often lead to the development of stereotypes and then usually to cultural misunderstandings, prejudices and also discrimination. Also, cultures are never static but are in a constant process of adaptation and change.

An important point in understanding the role of culture is that it must always be seen in its particular context. It may therefore be impossible to isolate 'pure' cultural beliefs and behaviour from the social and economic context in which they occur; for example, people may act in a particular way not because it is within their cultural tradition to do so but because they are simply too poor to do otherwise. Therefore in understanding health and illness, it is important to avoid 'victim blaming' – that is, seeing the poor health of a population as the sole result of its culture – instead of looking also at the economic or social situations of the individual. Helman cites as an example the case of the Black Report (Townsend & Davidson 1982) which showed that in the UK, health could clearly be correlated with income. In the developing

Antiracism, multiculturalism and the third way

world too, whatever the local culture, poor health can usually be correlated with a low income, lack of food and water, the sanitation that people can afford and so on. Thus, culture should never be considered in a vacuum but only as one component of a complex mix of influences on what people believe and how they live their lives.

A final misuse of the concept of culture, especially in medical care, is that its influence may be overemphasised in interpreting how some people present their symptoms to health professionals. Symptoms or behaviour may be ascribed to the person's culture when they are really due to an underlying physical or mental disorder. This form of cultural essentialism which results in 'victim blaming' has been vehemently criticised by the antiracist lobby, as we shall see in the following section.

THE ANTIRACIST EXPLANATION

Minority ethnic groups face discrimination at many levels in society. Ahmad (1993a, 1995), Pearson (1983), Donovan (1986) and Sheldon & Parker (1992) see cultural analysis as a diversion from the more important issue of racism. Racism may be seen as leading to disadvantage and inevitably to a higher rate of ill health (Benzeval et al 1995). Brah (1992), arguing against a cultural analysis, has stated that this is largely independent of other social experiences centred around class, gender, racism or sexuality, whilst Rattansi (1992) and Gilroy (1992) refer to the absence of these variables from the antiracist analysis too. This has led to the misconception that a group identified as culturally different is assumed to be internally homogeneous. Ahmad (1996) asserts that the rigid conception of culture emphasises cultural difference and helps to obscure the similarities between broadly defined cultural groups and the diversity within a cultural group. He goes on to say that discourses built around the concept of culture and cultural difference play an important part within the strategies of control of black people's lives through the state systems of immigration control, education, professional ideologies and practices.

Goldberg (1993) argues that 'ethnic reduction' – a repercussion of the multicultural position – first constructs all ethnic minorities as similar; they represent the 'other' but the 'other' is then disaggregated as some are seen as making progress towards assimilation while others are blamed for failing to do so. In this way the culture of the group is pathologised. Thus the 'other' points to elements of

Diversity and inequality in health care

lifestyle which differ from what is assumed to be a 'normal' British lifestyle (Ahmad 1993b, Donovan 1986, Pearson 1983, Pfeffer & Moynihan 1996, Sashidharan & Francis 1993, Senior & Bhopal 1994). Antiracists, such as Ahmad (1993b) have criticised the multiculturalists, such as Qureshi (1989), Healy & Aslam (1990) and Rack (1990), for contributing to the establishment of a deterministic link between the culture of minority ethnic groups and their morbidity, mortality and health behaviour. Ahmad (1993b), characteristically, calls them 'cultural merchants'.

Lambert & Sevak (1996) questioned the assumption made by multiculturalists that 'culture differences' in the UK population are predictably correlated with ethnic identification which affects health status, health-related behaviour and receptivity to health information. They have argued that cultural difference may have limited value in explaining differentials in health status, health beliefs and health-related behaviour in a multiethnic society. They cited Crawford (1977) who suggested that the emphasis placed on behavioural or 'lifestyle' factors to explain the high incidence of chronic conditions results in 'blaming the victim' while ignoring the social economic determinants of ill health. Ahmad (1996) has argued that the adherence to cultural explanations and its consequence of victim blaming constructs minority communities as dangerous to their own health. As was discussed in the previous section, the multiculturalist solution is to equip health providers with cultural understanding while at the same time, according to the antiracists, resocialising the culturally deviant through health education on the proper use of health services. Therefore, Mercer (1986) and Ahmad (1993a, 1996) suggest that by pathologising culture, we are making it the cause of as well as the solution to inequalities in health and health care.

Antiracism in the health service is not a strong or long tradition. Ahmad (1996) has suggested that the most important struggles in the area of 'race' and health are developments in the field of psychiatry, where black health workers and patients' groups have made a significant impact and have succeeded in challenging psychiatric orthodoxies. He cites the work of Mercer (1986), Fernando (1991) and Sashidharan & Francis (1993), as well as the contribution of the African-Caribbean Mental Health Association and the Confederation of Indian Organisations.

The antiracist health perspective is rooted in the history of black people, their experiences of colonisation, slavery and white domination. Indeed, the antiracists would argue that the health status of black people cannot be understood outside this framework. Ahmad (1993a) has stated that:

Antiracism, multiculturalism and the third way

Racial inequalities in health are a part, and a consequence, of racial inequalities in substantive rights of citizenship. Equally, although the scope for reducing racial inequalities in health lies largely outside the NHS, the equity of health care provision is also of paramount importance. These struggles for equitable health and health care are essentially located in the wider struggles for equity and dignity which have been a part of black people's history. (p 214)

A NEW UNIFIED APPROACH: THE THIRD WAY

Both the multicultural and the antiracist explanations have recently been criticised. According to Kelleher (1996), the multiculturalists have failed to emphasise adequately this important point: that in relation to understanding how people perceive health and illness, we must recognise that culture is a dynamic entity which changes to incorporate fresh ideas and perspectives, as people develop new ways of responding to their environment. On the other hand, he argues that the antiracists have tended to ignore the small-scale developments in health care delivery and the gradual improvements in attitudes that have taken place.

McKenzie & Crowcroft (1994) have argued that the multiculturalist approach is problematic in relation to second- and third-generation people who have had considerable contact with the English culture, having been born and educated in England; they do, however, believe that even though such individuals may come to regard their occupation as important in terms of their identity, they may still cling to what Nagel (1994) describes as 'symbolic ethnicity'. Hall (1992) goes further and suggests that the postmodern subject has no fixed identity, as the fully unified, completed, secure and coherent identity is a fantasy; the reality is that we often have contradictory identities within us, which we use in different situations.

Rattansi (1992) insists on the centrality of culture to the understanding of race, though not in an essentialist version of either the multiculturalist or the antiracist movements. He argues that at one level, there are many differences and contradictions within the two movements, whilst at a deeper level there are fundamental similarities of conceptualisation and prescription between multiculturalism and antiracism which are flawed. Although both movements have made important contributions, his judgement is that their frameworks and policies share significant and disabling weaknesses. Both the multiculturalist and the antiracist approaches can result in cultural essentialism, for the former often collapses analysis and prescription into some form of ethnic essentialism while in the latter, cultural essentialism emerges, ironically enough, partly out of the denial of ethnicity, as this is marginalised due to an exclusive focus on the 'black struggle' issues.

According to Rattansi (1992), cultural essentialism at its core has begun to disintegrate. First, through an ethnic backlash from the British Afro-Caribbean and Asian communities which protested at the homogenisation of different histories, cultures, needs and aspirations, implied in the use of the singular category 'black'; second, it has become increasingly clear that the 'black' category can marginalise other British minorities. Greek and Turkish Cypriots, for example, Jewish people and the Irish have been unable to find a voice within a political and cultural space marked out as 'black'. The category, in other words, functioned both to include and exclude; in so doing it tended not to engage with the variety of British racisms, although it was never intended to deny the existence of other racisms. The third challenge has come about as a range of 'black' groups have begun to explore, construct and express identities not exhausted by the experience of and struggle against racism; thus, we witness the emergence of what Stuart Hall (1992) has dubbed 'new ethnicities' which represent complex intersections of sexuality, ethnicity and class, imaginatively constructed through representations which break decisively with a framework of positive and negative images. A new cultural politics of difference is emerging which overlays the older ethnic differences.

Gilroy (1992) reaches the same conclusion but through a different emphasis. In his view, an alternative framework is emerging as a direct reaction to the moralistic excesses practised in the name of antiracism. Not only has antiracism evolved as a dictatorial form particularly in the context of local government, but it has also served to trivialise and isolate the struggles against other political antagonisms such as the contradictions of social and economic inequalities, the struggles of women and that of other marginalised groups. Yet, in Britain today, 'race' cannot be understood or grasped if it is falsely divorced from all these other political processes and power struggles.

Rattansi (1992) concludes that:

> For these developments to be taken seriously, the multiculturalists will have to abandon their additive models of cultural pluralism and their continuing obsession with the old ethnicities. Antiracists, on the other hand, will have to move beyond their reductive conceptions of culture and their fear of cultural differences as

Antiracism, multiculturalism and the third way

simply a source of division and weakness in the struggle against racism. They need to acknowledge the political significance of questions of national culture and ethnic identity, and to grasp how these intersect with questions of 'race' and racism. They will also have to work through the consequences of other British racisms, especially towards Jewish people and the Irish, and the realignment of older Western-Islamic polarities in the context of the Rushdie scandal. (p 41)

It could be argued that the level and volume of discourse generated by the multiculturalists, the antiracists and those suggesting an alternative framework strongly indicates the importance of addressing the quality of life of people from minority ethnic groups and the need to understand not only the difficulties they face but also the contribution which they make, as they actively engage in many different ways to establish themselves as equal citizens of this country. Citizenship, as Marshall (1964) explained, involves civil, political and social rights, all of which speak against the subordination of one group of people to another. However, numerous studies in the field of health and social welfare have provided evidence that there exist many inequalities amongst citizens in Britain. The Black Report (Townsend & Davidson 1982) found that mortality rates for both men and women aged 35 years and over in occupational classes I and II had declined while those in classes IV and V showed little change or had deteriorated. It argued that social and economic factors such as income, work, environment, education, housing, transport and lifestyles all affect health and all favour the better off. The Independent Inquiry into Inequalities in Health (Acheson 1998) concluded that although the last 20 years have brought a marked increase in prosperity and substantial reductions in mortality to the people of Great Britain as a whole, the gap in health between those at the top and the bottom of the social scale has widened. These socioeconomic differentials are also important in explaining health inequalities between different ethnic groups.

Oliver & Heaton (1994) state that many groups, such as women, minority ethnic groups, homosexuals, people with disabilities and those who suffer extreme poverty, feel that they are 'second-class citizens'. Naturally these groups are not mutually exclusive, if we take as an example the case of the minority ethnic groups, Kushnick (1988) claimed that because of the racism experienced by many people from minority ethnic groups, their position in terms of their economic circumstances, life chances and health is likely to be similar but it is also very likely that their position would be worse than that of the majority of white people living in Britain.

Oppenheim & Harker (1996) report that unemployment (an important indicator of poverty which in turn is one of the main indicators of ill health) affects the most vulnerable people in society such as the unskilled, the disabled and people from minority ethnic groups. In 1994 the male unemployment rate for black people and other minority ethnic groups was 25%, more than double the rate for white men which stood at 11%. The corresponding unemployment rates for women were 16% for black and minority ethnic women and only 7% for white women. For young men the unemployment rates of those from minority ethnic groups and white men was 37% versus 18%. For young women the figures were 27% and 12% respectively. Even with qualifications, members of minority ethnic groups are still more likely to experience unemployment because of discrimination. In 1994 the average hourly pay of all minority ethnic employees was 92% of that of white employees.

Oppenheim & Harker (1996) state that the persistence of a high level of poverty for black and minority ethnic groups is due to a number of factors:

- immigration policy which has curtailed access to welfare services
- inequalities in the labour market founded on deeply embedded discriminatory employment practices
- family patterns and the age structure of minority ethnic groups
- social security policies
- racism and discrimination in society as a whole.

In trying to analyse the determinants of health status, Benzeval et al (1992) modified Marmot et al's (1987) model of:

social forces → lifestyle and exposure differences → health differences.

They disaggregated 'social forces' into 'demographic and personal characteristics' and 'material, social and physical deprivation', all of which have both a direct and indirect influence on health status through their impact on lifestyle. Using data from the Health and Lifestyle Survey which were reported on by Blaxter (1990) and which they further analysed, Benzeval et al discuss the implications of age, gender, ethnicity, poverty, unemployment, housing, the environment, education, social isolation and social integration for lifestyle and health status. They concluded that on the basis of their findings, the links between deprivation and poor health had been clearly demonstrated and that they were certain that the

Antiracism, multiculturalism and the third way

distribution of health care resources ought to reflect the variations in social and economic circumstances in different geographical areas.

Whitehead (1995) suggests that four main policy levels seem to have emerged for tackling inequalities in health. These are: strengthening individuals, strengthening communities, improving access to essential facilities and services, and encouraging macro-economic and cultural change. It may be argued that these initiatives have become part of the NHS agenda, because of the consistent lobbying by the World Health Organization to persuade national and local governments to adopt the Health for All approach (WHO 1985), whose central aim is to ensure greater social equity in health by adopting policies which:

● reduce poverty in its widest sense
● secure the basic prerequisites for health for everybody – food, safe water, sanitation, decent housing and universal education
● ensure that everybody has access to effective health care.

So, in terms of the first policy level referred to by Whitehead (1995), individual strengthening policies, the aim is to build up a person's knowledge, motivation, competence and skills in order to enable him to alter his behaviour in relation to personal risk factors or to cope better with the stresses imposed by external health hazards. Strategies to promote personal empowerment would be very relevant to members of minority ethnic groups who, as discussed earlier, are more likely to be the victims of discrimination and social exclusion. The second policy level focuses on how people in disadvantaged communities can join together for mutual support which could strengthen the whole community against health hazards. Although the word 'community' is not clearly defined by Whitehead, reference is made to 'neighbourhoods'. The third policy level focuses on ensuring better access to what the WHO calls 'the prerequisites for health', whilst the fourth policy level aims at reducing poverty and the wider adverse effects of inequality in society. According to Whitehead, interventions at policy level 1 and 2 have tended to treat the symptoms rather than the underlying cause of the problem. As these have been discrete experiments or short-term projects, their overall impact on observed inequalities in health can only have been minimal. The challenge is to make the effective approaches more widespread and part of the mainstream services offered to people. In contrast, interventions at policy level 3 and 4 involve every section of the population and thus any improvements have the potential for benefiting everyone.

CONCLUSION

This chapter considered the arguments around the two predominant approaches to the health of minority ethnic groups: the multiculturalist and the antiracist. It went on to examine some of the current issues around the determinants of health and proposed an evolving unified approach, the strands of which seem to have found their way into the recent NHS reforms. Furthermore, the current NHS reforms aim to bring about a coordinated approach which will deal with all levels of policy and remove the fragmentation and bureaucracy of the internal market. In the introduction to *Partnerships in action: new opportunities for joint working between health and social services* (DoH 1998), the following key statement is made.

> The Government's strategic agenda is to work across boundaries to combat social exclusion, encourage welfare to work, tackle inequalities between men and women and other groups and improve the health in local communities. Both the White Paper *The new NHS: modern, dependable*, and the Green Paper *Our healthier nation – a contract for health* emphasised the need for effective working between the NHS and local authorities (both in their social services functions and more widely), underpinned by the new duty of partnership, and set in the strategic context of a local Health Improvement Programme. (p 5)

In terms of policy levels, the Green Paper identifies a number of layers and settings for action. First, the government level will help assess the risk to health by making sure that people are given accurate, understandable and credible information. Second, the health authorities will lead in the development of Health Improvement Programmes. Third, the local authorities will have a duty to promote the economic, social and environmental well-being of their areas. Fourth, businesses can bring new skills to bear, as well as improving the health and safety of their own employees. Fifth, voluntary bodies can act as advocates to give a powerful voice to local people. Sixth, individuals can take responsibility for their own health.

Three settings are identified: the healthy school which focuses on children, the healthy workplace which focuses on adults and the

Antiracism, multiculturalism and the third way

healthy neighbourhood which focuses on older people. Nurses have a very important role to play in all these settings. For example, most of us are familiar with the school nurse. However, the Acheson Report (1998) identifies three priorities which relate to schools and which should involve a greater role for the school nurse:

- the promotion of life management skills such as communication, coping with emotions and parenthood skills
- the delivery of more effective programmes to tackle substance misuse such as programmes which recognise the specific needs of the individual and the differing social and cultural contexts in which substance misuse is engendered, initiated and maintained
- the delivery of more effective sex education programmes which are tailored to the needs of the group they are intended to serve.

It appears that the emerging new approach – the third way – has integrated the health needs of minority ethnic groups within a broader agenda which is centred around the eradication of inequalities and the promotion of citizenship rights, responsibilities and involvement. Coote (1992) puts forwards the idea that life chances are closely linked to the idea of individual empowerment as a requirement of citizenship. This implies that all citizens must have equal access to services to ensure equal chances in life and thus the absence of unfair discrimination. It is too early to judge whether the government's 'third way', which is claimed to be between the old victim blaming (an approach linked to the previous Conservative government as well as with multiculturalism) and the nanny state of social engineering (associated with 'old Labour'), will positively affect the health of people from minority ethnic groups.

Practice checklist

Readers should consider the following issues which may inform practice.

- Consider your practice in terms of the three approaches that were presented in this chapter. Which approach is more akin to your current practice?
- Reflect on any actions you have taken or are planning to take in order to respond to the recommendations put forward by the Acheson Report (1998).

Discussion questions

- What is your view of the 'third way'? Is it possible to achieve the ambitious and integrated programme put forward by the government without any specific focus on 'racism'?
- 'Institutional racism' is very much alive according to the debates which followed the Stephen Lawrence inquiry and the publication of the Macpherson Report (1999). How is this currently manifested in your institution? What, if any, progress has been made?
- It could be argued that the nursing profession is a very powerful one because of its size and the central role it occupies within the NHS. Do you think that nurses are using this power to promote equality within the NHS? Give some positive and negative examples.

References

Acheson D (Chair) 1998 Independent inquiry into inequalities in health report. Stationery Office, London

Ahmad W I U 1993a Promoting equitable health and health care: a case for action. In: Ahmad W I U (ed) 'Race' and health in contemporary Britain. Open University Press, Buckingham

Ahmad W I U 1993b Making black people sick: 'race', ideology and health research. In: Ahmad W I U (ed) 'Race' and health in contemporary Britain. Open University Press, Buckingham

Ahmad W I U 1995 Review article: race and health. Sociology of Health and Illness 17(3):418–429

Ahmad W I U 1996 The trouble with culture. In: Kelleher D, Hillier S (eds) Researching cultural difference in health. Routledge, London

Anderson J, Elfert H, Lai M 1989 Ideology in the clinical context: chronic illness, ethnicity and the discourse on normalisation. Sociology of Health and Illness 11(3):253–278

Anthias F, Yuval-Davis N 1992 Racialized boundaries: race, nation, colour and class and the anti-racist struggle. Routledge, London

Audit Commission 1992 Making time for patients. HMSO, London

Benzeval M, Judge K, Solomon M 1992 Health status of Londoners. A comparative perspective. King's Fund, London

Benzeval M, Judge K, Whitehead M (eds) 1995 Tackling inequalities in health. An agenda for action. King's Fund, London

Blaxter M 1990 Health and lifestyles. Tavistock/Routledge, London

Brah A 1992 Difference, diversity and differentiation. In: Donald J, Rattansi A (eds) Race, culture and difference. Sage/Open University, London

Bulmer M 1986 Race and ethnicity. In: Burgess R G (ed) Key variables in social investigation. Routledge and Kegan Paul, London

Antiracism, multiculturalism and the third way

Coote A (ed) 1992 The welfare of citizens. Developing new social rights. IPPR/Rivers Oram Press, London

Crawford R 1977 You are dangerous to your health: the ideology and politics of victim blaming. International Journal of Health Services 7(4):663–680

Crowley J, Simmons S 1992 Mental health, race and ethnicity: a retrospective study of the care of ethnic minorities and whites in a psychiatric unit. Journal of Advanced Nursing 17:1078–1087

Currer C 1986 Concepts of mental well- and ill-being: the case of Pathan mothers in Britain. In: Currer C, Stacey M (eds) Concepts of health, illness and disease. Berg, Oxford

Department of Health 1998 Partnerships in action: new opportunities for joint working between health and social services. Stationery Office, London

Dobson S 1991 Transcultural nursing. Scutari Press, London

Donovan J L 1986 We don't buy sickness, it just comes. Health, illness and health care in the lives of black people in London. Gower, Aldershot

Fenton S 1985 Race, health and welfare. University of Bristol, Bristol

Fernando S 1991 Mental health, race and culture. Macmillan/MIND Publications, London

Francis E, David J, Johnson N, Sashidharan S D 1989 Black people and psychiatry in the UK. Psychiatric Bulletin 13:482–485

Gilroy P 1992 The end of antiracism. In: Donald J, Rattansi A (eds) Race, culture and difference. Sage/Open University, London

Goldberg D 1993 Racist culture. Blackwell, Oxford

Hall S 1992 New ethnicities. In: Donald J, Rattansi A (eds) Race, culture and difference. Sage/Open University, London

Healy M A, Aslam M 1990 The Asian community: medicines and traditions. Silver Link Publishing, Nottingham

Helman C G 1990 Culture, health and illness, 2nd edn. Butterworth Heinemann, Oxford

Kavanagh K H, Kennedy P H 1992 Promoting cultural diversity. Strategies for health care professionals. Sage, Newbury Park

Kelleher D 1996 A defence of the use of the terms 'ethnicity' and 'culture'. In: Kelleher D, Hillier S (eds) Researching cultural difference in health. Routledge, London

Kessing R M 1981 Cultural anthropology: a contemporary perspective. Holt, Rinehart and Winston, New York

King's Fund 1990 Racial equality: the nursing profession. Task Force Position Paper. Equal Opportunities Task Force Occasional Paper No 6. King's Fund Publishing Office, London

Kleinman A 1987 Anthropology and psychiatry: the role of culture in cross-cultural research on illness. British Journal of Psychiatry 151:447–454

Kushnick L 1988 Racism, the National Health Service and the health of black people. International Journal of Health Services 18(3):457–470

Lambert H, Sevak L 1996 Is 'cultural difference' a useful concept? Perceptions of health and the sources of ill health among Londoners of South Asian origin. In: Kelleher D, Hillier S (eds) Researching cultural difference in health. Routledge, London

LaVeist T 1993 Segregation, poverty and empowerment: health consequences for African Americans. Milbank Quarterly 71(1):41–64

Leach E 1982 Social anthropology. Fontana, Glasgow

Leininger M M 1978 Transcultural nursing: concepts, theories and practices. John Wiley, New York

Leininger M M 1991 (ed) Culture care, diversity and universality: a theory of nursing. NLN Press, New York

Leininger M M 1995 Transcultural nursing. Concepts, theories, research and practices, 2nd edn. McGraw-Hill, New York

Levin J 1994a Religion and health: is there an association, is it valid, and is it causal? Social Science and Medicine 38(11):1475–1482

Levin J 1994b Religion in aging and health. Sage, London

Macpherson W (Chair) 1999 The Stephen Lawrence inquiry. Stationery Office, London

Marmot M, Kogevinas M, Elston M 1987 Social/economic status and disease. Annual Review of Public Health 8:111–135

Marshall T H 1964 Citizenship and social class. In: Marshall T H (ed) Class, citizenship and social development. Doubleday, New York

McKenzie K J, Crowcroft N S 1994 Race, ethnicity, culture, and science. British Medical Journal 309:286–287

McNaught A 1987 Health action and ethnic minorities. National Community Health Resource and Bedford Square Press, London

Mercer K 1986 Racism and transcultural psychiatry. In: Millar P, Rose N (eds) The power of psychiatry. Polity Press, London

Nagel J 1994 Constructing ethnicity: creating and recreating ethnic identity and culture. Social Problems 41(1):152–176

Oliver D, Heaton D 1994 The foundations of citizenship. Harvester Wheatsheaf, London

Oppenheim C, Harker L 1996 Poverty, the facts, 3rd edn. Child Poverty Action Group, London

Pearson M 1983 The politics of ethnic minority health studies. Radical Community Medicine 16:34–44

Pfeffer N, Moynihan C 1996 Ethnicity and health beliefs with respect to cancer: a critical review of methodology. British Journal of Cancer 74 (Suppl. XXIX): S66–S72

Qureshi B 1989 Transcultural medicine. Kluwer Academic, Dordrecht

Rack P 1990 Psychological and psychiatric disorders. In: McAvoy B, Donaldson L (eds) Health care for Asians. Oxford University Press, Oxford

Rattansi A 1992 Changing the subject? Racism, culture and education. In: Donald J, Rattansi A (eds) Race, culture and difference. Sage/Open University, London

Sashidharan S, Francis E 1993 Epidemiology, ethnicity and schizophrenia. In: Ahmad W I U (ed) 'Race' and health in contemporary Britain. Open University Press, Buckingham

Senior P, Bhopal R 1994 Ethnicity as a variable in epidemiological research. British Medical Journal 309:327–330

Sheldon T A, Parker H 1992 Race and ethnicity in health research. Journal of Public Health Medicine 14(2):104–110

Antiracism, multiculturalism and the third way

Smaje C 1995 Health, 'race' and ethnicity. Making sense of the evidence. King's Fund Institute, London

Spector R E 1991 Cultural diversity in health and illness, 3rd edn. Appleton and Lange, Norwalk

Torkington P 1984 The racist and sexist delivery of the NHS – the experience of black women. In: O'Sullivan S (ed) Womens' health, a Spare Rib reader. Pandora, London

Townsend P, Davidson N 1982 Inequalities in health: the Black Report. Penguin, Harmondsworth

Tylor E B 1871 Primitive culture: research into the development of mythology, philosophy, religion, art and customs. John Murray, London

Whitehead M 1995 Tackling inequalities: a review of policy initiatives. In: Benzeval M, Judge K, Whitehead M (eds) Tackling inequalities in health. An agenda for action. King's Fund, London

WHO 1985 Targets for Health for All by the Year 2000. WHO, Regional Office for Europe, Copenhagen

Further reading

Department of Health 1999 Reducing health inequalities: an action report. Stationery Office, London

Department of Health 1999 Making a difference. Strengthening the nursing, midwifery and health visiting contribution to health and healthcare. DoH, London

Department of Health 1999 Saving lives: our healthier nation. DoH, London

Macpherson W (Chair) 1999 The Stephen Lawrence inquiry. Stationery Office, London

NHSE 1998 Tackling racial harassment in the NHS. A plan for action. DoH, London

Papadopoulos I, Tilki M, Taylor G 1998 Transcultural care: a guide for health care professionals. Quay Books, Salisbury

Application **2:1**
Carol Baxter, Tina Moore

Valuing diversity and avoiding discrimination in the admission of ethnic minorities to nursing courses

INTRODUCTION

The fall in the supply of potential new recruits to the nursing labour force has occurred at the same time as an increased demand on the NHS. Increasing competition from the service sector for the same pool of female labour has compounded this staffing crisis facing the NHS. This set of circumstances has brought the potential labour supply for Britain's minority ethnic communities into sharper focus. The age profile of this section of the population is younger in comparison with the population as a whole; thus people born outside the UK represent a significant pool of potential young workers (OPCS 1993). In short, then, it has been widely recognised that if such groups are underrepresented in the nursing, midwifery and health-visiting workforce, this would reflect a lack of equity and fairness as well as undermining the potential of the NHS to provide appropriate services to this section of the population (Iganski et al 1998).

More than a decade ago, Baxter (1987) warned that nursing was increasingly becoming an unattractive career for ethnic minorities in the UK. This forecast was based on the premise of the pervasiveness and deterrent effect of racial discrimination in the NHS and was the first to alert the profession to this potential problem and the need for an equal opportunities strategy. Lee-Cunin (1989) and Beishon et al (1995) also pointed to the prevalence of racism in the health service in relation to nurses. A subsequent research project commissioned by the English National Board used quantitative and qualitative approaches to evaluate the implementation of the Board's equal opportunities policy (Iganski et al 1998). The findings described applications from members of ethnic minority groups to preregistration nursing and midwifery training as 'a complex pattern of under- and in some cases overrepresentation'. More recently, there has been a notable increase in the number of overseas students (Castledine 2000).

The following scenarios (based on recent real-life experiences) nevertheless demonstrate how other areas of discrimination can still pose problems of access to nurse education for ethnic minority applicants.

Case study 2.1.1   Monica

Monica, a 54-year-old enrolled nurse from the Caribbean, has 36 years nursing experience in England. She has never left the profession and opted to work on a part-time basis whilst bringing up a family.

During an appraisal with her manager, it became evident that Monica was showing the potential to be an effective first-level nurse. The possibility of her undertaking a conversion course to first-level registration was discussed. After thoughtful consideration Monica decided that she was ready to undertake such a course and prepared herself by undertaking various in-house study sessions and kept up to date by reading journals on a regular basis. This was evidenced in her professional portfolio of achievements.

She applied to do the course at her local university. At interview a point was made about her age. She was specifically asked why she had not applied for the course much earlier, implying that her age may prove to be problematic. She was also asked how she would cope with the academic demands of the course and her feelings in relation to being in a classroom with predominantly younger students.

Reflecting upon the experience of the interview, Monica felt that it did not go well for her. She not was surprised when she received a letter stating that she was unsuccessful in getting a place. However, feeling demoralised, she did not investigate the reasons why. She also gave up all hope of becoming a first-level nurse.

Diversity and inequality in health care

Case study 2.1.2 Lisa

Lisa, a 20-year-old Italian, has lived in England with relatives for 2 years. She speaks fluent English with a strong Italian accent. From an early age Lisa had wanted to be a nurse and had achieved the necessary grades (including the equivalent of a GCSE Grade A in English) required for entry to nurse education in the UK.

Convinced that universities in England offered the best education and experience, she made applications to several universities and was successful in gaining one interview. During the interview she was asked about her Italian culture and if she felt it would inhibit her in any way. At the end of the interview, she was informed that she would be required to take an oral and written English language test before selection could be completed.

On challenging this decision, Lisa was informed that it was standard procedure for all non-English-born students. She refused to sit the language test, claiming that there was no problem with her written and spoken language, as indicated by her qualifications. A few weeks later, she received notification that she had been unsuccessful in her application, as she failed to adhere to the policy that was currently in place. Lisa was not discouraged by this and continued to pursue her applications with other universities.

COMMENTARY

The factors of age and proficiency in English are the two obvious areas under consideration in these scenarios. Traditional recruitment approaches portrayed nurses as 18 years old, white, female and from the English upper social classes. Whilst this limited image of nurses is now being challenged, such attitudes still get in the way of fairness in the recruitment and selection process.

Age

It is appreciated that an important issue in recruitment and selection is whether it will be worth investing in training someone who is so close to retirement. Such cost implications, however, are often given priority over the wealth of life and professional experience which applicants have to offer. For example, in the 1980s and early 1990s many organisations, faced with the need to reduce the size of their workforce, used age as an 'easy to apply' criterion for selecting people for redundancy. Subsequently, they discovered that key skills, knowledge, information and corporate memory had been lost from the organisation (DfEE 1999).

Admission of ethnic minorities to nursing courses

65

In the context of the classroom, preoccupation with the mature applicant's ability to learn new skills can result in the positive contribution which their higher levels of motivation can have in enhancing group learning being overlooked. Whereas there may not be an upper age limit set by institutions for admission to courses, interviewers can be forced to introduce age as an arbitrary sifting measure, based on age stereotypes such as 'You can't teach an old dog new tricks'. Many employers have found that this is not true. Many older workers who lost their jobs in the 1980s and early 1990s have successfully moved into new careers (Barclays Bank 1998). In assessing applicant's ability, objective performance assessments and dialogue and discussion are alternatives to age which can give employers and individuals the best indication of when the time may be right to change working patterns.

Age diversity is about selecting the best person, regardless of age. This applies to investing in the continuing professional development and the skills of older nurses. A key government initiative which will help to achieve age diversity is the recent ministerial group set up to develop a government strategy for older people. This aims to ensure that policy affecting older people (50 and over) is effectively coordinated and takes account of their needs (DFEE 1999).

Proficiency in English

The accent and syntax commonly used by people who do not speak English as a first language can conjure up the stereotypical image of the 'foreigner who is unable to speak and understand English'. However, many second-language English speakers are also bi- or even multilingual, an attribute less commonly found amongst native English speakers. It is interesting to note that the usual mechanisms for considering applicants whose previous training was given in a language other than English or where English was not the official language of the country in which the training was undertaken is that the applicant is required to demonstrate proficiency in English by achieving a high score in the examination set by the International English Language Testing Service. This policy should be challenged, however, since it is open to indiscriminate use. Furthermore, over the past 5–10 years it has become increasingly obvious to the UKCC that some foreign applicants for general nurse registration in the UK meet or exceed the educational requirements for registration in this country (Castledine 2000).

Indirect racial discrimination

On the surface it would appear that these scenarios are simply discussing proficiency in English and age discrimination but the reality is more complex. Discrimination in these areas can inadvertently result in discrimination on racial grounds. By this it is meant that a particular criterion (age and proficiency in English in this context) applies equally to all but has the effect of disadvantaging one particular section of the population. Ethnic minority applicants to nurse education are more likely to find themselves in the circumstances described above than their white counterparts. It is well recognised, for example, that they are overrepresented on the roll as compared to the register of nurses, have less access to conversion courses than their white counterparts and wait much longer to get on to such courses (Akinsanya 1988, Baxter 1987, Beishon et al 1995, King's Fund 1990). Hence, many will be at the older end of the age spectrum by the time they are able to convert. Similarly, the increasing numbers of overseas recruits are more likely to speak with 'foreign accents' which increases the risk of their communication skills and competence in English being wrongly called into question.

Added value

Discrimination of this nature is not only unfair but can also be short-sighted because it can restrict the potential of the nursing profession. People such as Monica and Lisa can bring unique views and specific knowledge to nursing. They have additional skills which would be useful in providing culturally appropriate care. Furthermore, a diverse mix of the staff in clinical settings can be an educational advantage for home students who could learn by example to do likewise. Dores (1993) pointed out that as nursing is a profession that serves a diverse society, diversity in recruitment is a desirable goal.

A fair and effective recruitment process requires a comprehensive effort that integrates attitudes, values, content and actions and involves all aspects of the educational system simultaneously. Diversity relates to people and their unique experiences and requires the creation of an environment where none is advantaged or disadvantaged by prejudices and biases and where every person is encouraged to fully utilise their unique talents, skills, abilities and experiences.

The interview remains the most commonly used means of selection. All those involved should have training which not only covers interviewing techniques but also equal opportunities aspects of selection. Interviewers must not only be aware of the need to ask job/course-related questions but also avoid basing selection decisions on bias and stereotypes. They will also need to be mindful of the Royal College of Nursing guidelines *Equality in education*, an extract from which is outlined below (RCN 1995).

ROYAL COLLEGE GUIDELINES ON EQUALITY IN EDUCATION

The RCN guidelines on equality in education aim to give practical guidance to help nurses understand their rights to equal treatment in selection and recruitment to nursing education courses. They also aim to demonstrate to nursing educators how policies can be implemented and accessed to eliminate discrimination and enhance equality of opportunity.

They are based on two areas of concern. First, that recruitment/admission criteria and procedures vary both within and between colleges of nursing, faculties, departments and courses and may stipulate different academic requirements and apply a variety of non-academic criteria. Second, that a wide variety of methods of selection or assessment are being used to evaluate progress, attainment and aptitude.

The RCN identified that some methods of assessment will be formal tests and examinations. Others may be informal and involve subjective evaluations by tutors and others. All are important in determining access to, and exclusion from, educational opportunities and may also have a significant bearing on subsequent career and work opportunities. It stipulated that applicants may have non-academic skills, talents and experience which enhance their suitability for admissions to courses. Previous employment history, life experience and management skills are examples of positive non-academic criteria.

The guidelines identify a number of actions which would be discriminatory, as follows:

Recruitment/admissions

- Requiring students to have academic qualifications which exceeded the knowledge and skills needed to undertake the course, if these requirements cannot be shown to be justifiable.
- Applying non-academic criteria in determining admission to courses if they cannot be shown to be justified. Placing emphasis on factors such as family connections, appearance, communication skills, attitudes, cultural interests, all of which may have the effect of excluding disproportionate numbers of candidates from particular groups.
- Imposing quotas, for instance to achieve 'balance' in relation to gender, race and disability.
- Stipulating uniform and dress regulations that result in the rejection of a student who cannot comply for cultural or religious reasons. For example, a requirement that women nursing

students must wear dresses could exclude a high proportion of Muslims who wish to follow their religious requirement to cover their legs.
- Refusing a student admission to a course on the grounds of race, sex or marital status or to expect them to have better qualifications than others because of these grounds.

Selection/assessments

- Applying criteria or procedures which are culturally biased (that is, they assume a uniformity in cultural, linguistic, religious and lifestyle experiences and result in a lower assessment being given to a disproportionately higher number of students from particular groups) if those requirements cannot be justified.
- Giving students lower assessments on grounds of race, gender, disability or sexuality, based on assumptions (conscious or unconscious) about the relative abilities and characteristics of different groups.
- Including biased comments based on racial origins, gender, sexuality or disability on student records of achievement/reports.
- Allocating particular types of courses on racial or gender grounds. Discrimination would occur if a disproportionately higher number of students from particular groups were placed in lower graded courses if this could not be justified on educational grounds.

The RCN also gave examples of some positive steps which have been taken by many educational establishments and employers to encourage participation by particular groups where there is under-representation, such as:

- monitoring admissions by gender, disability and ethnicity and taking remedial action where underrepresentation occurs
- advertising courses in the ethnic minority or gay press or magazines aimed at women
- encouraging women or particular minority groups to apply for courses where there is underrepresentation
- including equality statements in guidance and information documents on nursing courses, such as the English National Board Applicant Handbook
- ensuring that tests and examinations are free of cultural bias. In particular, the design and use of psychometric tests for recruitment and assessment may affect equality of opportunity for people from minority groups
- setting targets on grounds of race, sex and disability where there is underrepresentation of particular groups
- recording on a student's report or record of achievement if the student had been a victim of racial or sexual harassment, since this might have a bearing on motivation and attainment.

Admission of ethnic minorities to nursing courses

References

Akinsanya J 1988 Ethnic minority nurses, midwives and health visitors: what role for them in the National Health Service? New Community 14:444–450

Barclays Bank 1998 Small business review on the third age entrepreneurs. Barclays Bank, London

Baxter C 1987 The black nurses: an endangered species. A case for equal opportunities in nursing. National Extension College, Cambridge

Beishon S, Virdee S, Hagell A 1995 Nursing in a multi-ethnic NHS. Policy Studies Institute, London

Castledine G 2000 Accepting the diversity of overseas nurses. British Journal of Nursing 9(13):886

Department for Education and Employment 1999 Age diversity in employment: a code of practice. Department for Education and Employment, Nottingham

Dores N S 1993 Effects of a participative intervention on high school students. Image and valuation of nursing. Journal of Professional Nursing 9(1):41–49

Iganski P, Mason D, Humphries A, Watkins M 1998 The black nurse: ever an endangered species? Nursing Times Research 3(5):325–338

King's Fund Equal Opportunities Task Force 1990 Racial equality: the nursing profession. Equal Opportunities Task Force Occasional Paper No. 6. King's Fund, London

Lee-Cunin M 1989 Daughters of Seacole. A study of black nurses in West Yorkshire. West Yorkshire Low Pay Unit, Batley

OPCS 1993 1991 census: ethnic group and country of birth. Great Britain. Volume 2. HMSO, London

RCN 1995 Equality in education (pamphlet). RCN, London

Further reading

Ludlow R, Panton F 1991 Discrimination in recruitment: the essence of successful staff selection. Prentice Hall, London

Chapter **Three**

Women in the caring professions: a case in point

Joy Foster

OVERVIEW

The purpose of this chapter is to encourage readers to reflect on issues of gender within their organisations. It explores issues relating to the position of women and men in the workforce using historical snapshots to illustrate parallels between health and social service settings. The chapter challenges readers to reflect on their own expectations in relation to the roles and appropriate behaviour ascribed to women and men and to consider various explanations for the inequitable distribution of women and men within organisations. It draws attention to the importance for both women and men managers of challenging stereotypes, in order to fully utilise the skills and abilities of the workforce and to enable its members to realise their potential. Finally, it suggests that there are benefits for both women and men in redefining traditional roles and facilitating a balance between responsibilities in the public and domestic spheres.

Objectives

This chapter explores the following themes and issues:
- the gendered structure of organisations in health and social care in historical and contemporary contexts
- gendered roles and stereotyping
- the legitimacy of women in management in health and social care
- structural discrimination.

INTRODUCTION

Access to management in all large organisations is mediated by gender and despite the overwhelming dominance of women as employees in health and social care, the large organisations for which they work conform to the common gender structure. In both spheres the organisational management is dominated at senior levels by men, predominantly white men. The organisational structures and the beliefs of managers within them tend to perpetuate inequality. The historical snapshots which follow illustrate the importance of ideology in defining the appropriate activities of women and men and in perpetuating the gender divisions in organisations. But first let us consider the position at the start of the 21st century.

THE CURRENT POSITION

In a number of ways the caring professions, in particular nursing and social work, can be viewed as a success story for women. By increasing the availability of paid employment for women during the late 19th and 20th centuries, the growth in these occupations made economic independence a possibility for many. As we approached the millennium, the majority of employees in both the health service and in social work in England were women (see Box 3.1). The majority of their clients are also women. Both occupations have faced difficulties in gaining professional status, arguably precisely because they have a predominantly female workforce (see, e.g., Witz 1992), and in both occupations the positions of power and authority are disproportionately held by men. Women throughout the labour force are concentrated in certain types of occupation; that is, they are segregated horizontally into areas such as catering, cleaning, clerical and caring roles. Women also have restricted access to the higher levels of most organisations, that is, they are segregated vertically, with higher proportions of women at the lower levels of organisations. Even in health and social services organisations, which employ unusually high proportions of women, the patterns of horizontal and vertical segregation are reproduced.

In the late 1980s, full-time women nurses and midwives in the NHS outnumbered full-time men by nearly six to one. Part-time

Diversity and inequality in health care

> **Box 3.1**   Gender distribution in the NHS 1988–89
>
> *Nurses and Midwives*
>
> | Women full time | Men full time | Women part time | Men part time | Total women | Total men |
> |---|---|---|---|---|---|
> | 309 871 | 53 517 | 220 534 | 4 297 | 530 405 | 57 814 |
>
> *General and Senior Managers*
>
> | Women full time | Men full time |
> |---|---|
> | 239 | 1154 |
>
> *Source*: Equal Opportunities Commission 1991

women outnumbered part-time men by over 51 to one. Women also dominated a number of other occupational groupings in the NHS, notably professions allied to medicine and administrative and clerical officers. However, the figures for general and senior managers for the same year, 1988–89, show a very different gender distribution in the management of the health service (see Box 3.1). Whilst there were over 1100 men (1154) identified as managers and working full time, there were only 254 women. The numbers of managers working part time was negligible. Men therefore outnumbered women as managers in the health service by almost five to one.

The ethnic origins of staff are not recorded within the EOC (1991) report but elsewhere (Beishon et al 1995), figures have been presented to show that some 6.3% of female nurses came from minority ethnic groups (compared with 3.6% of all females in employment) and that 14.7% of male nurses belonged to minority ethnic groups (compared with 3.9% of all males in employment). The health service is therefore a significant employer of members of minority ethnic groups.

A similar gender structure is to be found in social services departments. These organisations are the statutory providers of social care. They are the largest departments within local authorities and employ some 350 000 people in England and Wales, of whom 86% are women (Nottage 1991). Despite this, in 1990 80% of the directors of social services in England were men and seven of the eight departments in Wales were headed by men. There were at least two black men directors but of the 20% of directors who were women, all were white.

It is clear therefore that the workforce of both the NHS and of social services departments in the late 1980s continued to be numerically dominated by women but hierarchically dominated

Women in the caring professions

by men. There is no evidence to indicate any significant change in the course of the last decade and the occupations share interesting parallels currently and historically.

THE HISTORICAL DEVELOPMENT OF NURSING AND SOCIAL WORK

The histories of nursing and social work show both similarities and differences. A comprehensive review of these is beyond the scope of this chapter but a sense can be gained by exploring three historical snapshots drawn around the mid-19th to early 20th-century origins of the occupations, the period in the 1940s and 1950s when the welfare state was established and the NHS came into being and the reforms of the late 1960s and early 1970s. These three periods illustrate the importance of ideological factors in defining suitable work for women (and men). The focus in each period is nursing within the context of the hospital and women in statutory social work organisations since these are the major employment arenas for the occupations.

The late 19th and early 20th centuries

The social changes which accompanied the industrial revolution included the rapid emergence of new occupations, rapid urbanisation and concerns, whether humanitarian or otherwise, about the health and social conditions of the population. The late 19th-century strivings of women, including their struggles to gain access to universities and to gain the vote, were happening during a period when the opportunities for employment for women remained very restricted. Nursing and social work were recognised by advocates of women's progress as presenting opportunities for women, at a time when the roles considered appropriate for women were highly circumscribed. However, despite opening up opportunities for women, the occupations have developed in ways which reinforced rather than undermined the patriarchal structure of society and the reinforcement of patriarchal ideology has been an important feature of the way in which both nursing and social work have developed.

The assumptions which take men as the norm and measure women against them underpin the patriarchal structure of our society and perpetuate the power imbalance between women and men. There is a remarkable degree of historical continuity in ideology which explains differences in the societal locations of women and men as being the inevitable result of biological differences.

In late Victorian society, nursing and social work were both regarded as being suited to women's innate and biologically determined characteristics. The association of 'caring' with women is nowhere more evident than in their involvement in the 'caring' occupations. The development of employment opportunities in nursing and social work was accompanied by explanations that these were areas of work appropriate for women because they were extensions of their domestic role which in itself was founded on 'natural laws'.

In her preface to *Women's Work* published in 1894, Lady Dilke refers to the 'operation of natural laws' as follows:

> If we attempt to ignore these laws, we are at once landed in a sea of difficulties. Take the very question of 'Women's Work'. At the outset we are brought face to face with facts which show us that all employments are not equally suitable to men and women. We find that, in the case of mothers at least, there are many occupations for which they are wholly unfit but in which men may engage with impunity. (Dilke & Whitley 1894)

Particularly during the late 19th century, the medical profession itself played a significant part in providing an ideological justification for the sexual division of labour (see, e.g., Doyal & Elston 1986). As women sought access to universities and via them to the medical profession, efforts were made to exclude them on the basis that intellectual activity was dangerous for women. This was presented as a moral argument and as resulting from a concern for women's health.

> The cost of activity, and especially of cerebral activity, which is very costly, has to be met ... The reproductive capacity is diminished in various degrees sometimes to the extent of inability to bear children, more frequently to the extent of inability to yield milk, and in numerous cases to a smaller extent which I must leave unspecified. (Herbert Spencer 1904, *The principles of ethics,* cited in Stibbs 1992)

As Doyal & Elston (1986) point out, the medical model of women has had a pervasive influence on societal perceptions and is itself underpinned by assumptions which are rarely made explicit. These assumptions reflect deeply held traditions and values in relation to the sexes. They explain that the taken-for-granted assumption in many medical textbooks is that:

> ...men are 'normal' whereas women are 'abnormal' and ... this abnormality stems from the fact that women's natural role is motherhood. (p 180)

Women in the caring professions

Six Steps to **Effective Management**

By the late 19th century nursing had 'the classic contours of a woman's occupation, overcrowding, stagnating wages, uncontrolled entry and varying standards of training' (Harrison 1996).

Dilke & Whitley (1894) noted that:

> Nurses are supposed to take it up in a missionary spirit for the good of the community without regard to their own comfort or health. Now unfortunately the more 'noble' a profession is considered the greater is the tendency to neglect the material well being of those concerned in it and nurses have reason to feel full force of this misplaced sentiment. (p 28)

The emergence of nursing as a paid occupation was arguably a result of the development of hospitals and the growth of medicine as a scientifically based activity. However, from its inception this paid activity was a poorly paid activity and the role of the nurse was secondary and subservient to that of the doctor. The patriarchal relationships between women and men were not threatened by an arrangement of this kind with the power distribution and roles reinforcing and being reinforced by the patterns elsewhere in society (Gamarnikou 1978, Kuhn & Wolpe 1978).

However, it should not be assumed that women were satisfied with this situation. The introduction of training and education for nurses was seen as necessary if the power over nursing itself was to be taken out of the hands of men. Women sought to improve their control over this particular occupation, without challenging either its association with women or the underlying stereotypes and biological determinism which this association reflected. For example, Florence Nightingale seems to have been optimistic that nursing would have a distinctive role to play in health care. But she saw it as specifically 'women's work' and considered that women should control their own sphere, but should not challenge the role and decisions of doctors who were generally male. The association of medicine with treatment and curing and of these with doctors and men sits alongside an association of nursing with caring and women and is rooted in 19th-century attitudes to women and men. It reflects, too, the restricted educational opportunities available to women. The emphasis on providing education for an occupation associated with women marked the beginning of a long process towards professionalisation which is also associated with a change in class orientation and aspirations for the occupation.

There was an expectation, however, that the management of nursing would be an integral part of the occupation rather than separate from it and Nightingale herself had much to say about these aspects of the occupation and the role of the matron (see Ulrich 1992). It was this role which attracted 'distressed gentlewomen' from the middle classes (Dingwall et al 1988) and those women who had experience of managing domestic servants. Nursing originally 'was an unskilled occupation drawn substantially from older women' (Doyal & Elston 1986, p 124) and 'something women did [and still do] in their homes' (p 196).

In the late 19th century social work was also presented as an extension of women's domestic role. The early advocates of social work within the Charity Organisation Society (COS) were mainly men, although the visitors carrying out the work were women, often of independent means and engaged in voluntary activity. The concept of women being paid for such activity, and indeed of their engaging in it, flew in the face of an expectation that middle-class women would be content managing their homes and domestic affairs. Whereas in the early history of nursing much of the work was of an 'institutional domestic' kind (Dale & Foster 1986, p 26) the COS visitor acted as an adviser, a role more akin to that of manager of the home or of domestic servants rather than representing an extension of a hands-on caring role. Both occupations shared a need for the support of upper-class women and men for their development and advancement but by the early 20th century both offered opportunities of paid employment to women on a scale not previously available.

After the Second World War: women as legitimate managers

Whilst both world wars were important in extending the employment of women, the period following the Second World War was particularly significant in the histories of both nursing and social work. Women were empowered by having been drawn into the workforce and into occupations from which they had previously been excluded. Towards the end of the Second World War many working women were taking a more militant stance on equal pay. In 1944 an Equal Pay Campaign Committee was set up with representatives from 100 women's organisations with a combined membership of no less than four million women (Dale & Foster 1986, p 19).

The same year saw the publication of the White Paper on a national health service, which came into effect in 1948. As a result of this a new regional system of hospital administration was established, with 14 regional hospital boards and 377 hospital management committees. The management of hospital services was at the heart of the reforms but in proposing and implementing the changes, little attention appears to have been given to the interests of nurses. Within the system of national professional advisory groups which was set up, even the Standing Nursing Advisory Committee had only a small majority of its members, 12 of the 22, drawn from the nursing profession (Dingwall et al 1988, p 108). With hindsight, it is interesting that the gender balance of the membership is not identified.

The establishment of the NHS put a particular spotlight on hospital services. Hospitals were significant organisations which required management and the operational management of hospitals was largely in the hands of women. The hospital matron was rarely male. The fact that little attention was paid to gender issues at the time may, ironically, have been beneficial for women. The lack of attention given to nursing and nurses may have facilitated a retention of authority and management in women's hands. The removal of this, the challenge to women's authority and capacity for management, was to come later.

Within social work the period after the Second World War also saw an initiative which enhanced the opportunities for women to access positions of authority. The establishment of children's departments, also in 1948, resulted in the emergence for the first time of significant numbers of women as chief officers in local government departments. This emergence stands in contrast to the rhetoric of the time which stressed the importance to women of marriage and childbearing. As Elizabeth Wilson writes of the time:

> What was continually emphasised was that, having won emancipation, women were rejecting it, and continued to put marriage and child rearing first. (Wilson 1977, p 60)

The contradiction was to some extent managed by emphasising the loss of young male lives during the war and the consequent need for women to earn their own living. Nevertheless, in both hospitals and children's departments the position of women presented a challenge to the usual associations of women with the private sphere of the home. Particularly significant is the fact that women occupied positions of authority in these occupations at this time. Hospital matrons and children's officers were involved in managing staff and in managing budgets and services. In both occupations the roles were significantly managerial. Despite this, in subsequent developments in the occupations and organisations, the managerial element of women's activities has been largely overlooked. The significance of this omission becomes evident only with the benefit of hindsight and a recognition of the importance of the emergence of management and managerialism in the later part of the century.

The challenge presented to the status quo by women in authority was reduced by a continued association of these spheres with specifically 'feminine' qualities. In the 1940s and 1950s, however, women turned such essentialist arguments about their 'special qualities' to their advantage and the emergence of children's departments provides an interesting illustration of this strategy. Children's departments were established on the recommendations of the Curtis Committee, chaired by Myra Curtis. In their report the committee used the pronoun 'she' throughout in referring to the chief officer of the new department. This was a departure from convention to which they made explicit reference, explaining that they were deliberately breaking with convention and using the feminine pronoun not because men should be excluded but because they felt that the qualities required in the post were more likely to be found in women. The report specified both desirable qualifications and personal characteristics.

> The Children's Officer should, in our view, be highly qualified academically, if possible be a graduate who also has a social science diploma. She should not be under thirty at the time of appointment and should have some experience of work with children. She should have marked administrative capacity and be able to work easily with local government committees.
>
> ...She should be genial and friendly in manner and able to set both children and adults at their ease.
> Curtis Report 1946 paragraph 446

Thus the committee utilised essentialist arguments about women's 'special qualities' to good effect. They argued that this was a task which required particular personal skills and qualities and took advantage of the association of caring, and in particular of caring for children, with women. The success of this strategy can be inferred from the numbers of women and men appointed initially to these posts for in 1948, of the 133 children's departments established, 96 were headed by women. The late 1940s and 1950s therefore were a period when women had achieved significant presence as children's officers in local government and as matrons of hospitals.

The late 1960s: the removal of women managers

Women's hold over positions of authority was to prove a tenuous one and subsequent developments, viewed with the benefits of hindsight, reveal the dangers inherent in accepting and working within biologically deterministic arguments. With hindsight we might argue that this was a dangerous strategy. If the objective was to retain power over their occupation in the hands of women, the strategy was initially successful but subsequently failed. The problems which adoption of this strategy subsequently presented for women can be traced to reforms affecting the two occupations in the late 1960s. In that decade, the Report of the Committee on Senior Nursing Staff Structure (the Salmon Report published in 1966) and the Report of the Committee on Local Authority and Allied Personal Social Services (the Seebohm Report published in 1968) were both followed by a change in the gender access to senior roles, the former in hospitals and the latter in local authority social work. The challenge which had been presented by women holding positions of authority was effectively countered by the reforms which ensued.

The Salmon Report 'introduced to nursing a new language, the language of management' (Watkin 1975, p 318), a language inherently associated with masculinity. Although the report expresses concern about a 'seeming inability on the part of nurses to assert the rights of their emergent profession' and sees a need for professional representation on governing bodies, the report marks an implicit attack on hospital matrons who *did* have the right to membership of these bodies. The attack was based partly on the range of size of hospitals which they might head and the consequent variety of the extent of their responsibilities. The committee recommended the use of the term 'nursing officer' which could be applied to male as well as female officers, retaining the title 'matron' only for women. The report also placed a particular emphasis on the need for 'managerial skills'.

> Nurses in top management need, most of all, well developed managerial skills ... Provided he or she has shown the proper managerial ability it does not matter the route to the top. (para 1.15, quoted in Watkin 1975, p 323)

The management of hospitals, a sphere of authority which had been primarily in the hands of women as matrons, was redefined. At the same time there was criticism of matrons who had sought to legitimise the idea of a female occupation and female authority and to 'preserve their occupational identity' (Dale & Foster 1986, p 28) as reflecting self-interest. Whether or not the Salmon reforms were a deliberate strategy to remove women from positions of authority, this was their effect and the reforms ensured that men had greater access to positions of control and women were removed from them. There was an eightfold increase in the numbers of men in the top two nursing grades between 1969 and 1972 compared with only a fivefold increase in the numbers of women so that by 1972 men occupied a third of the posts at these levels (Carpenter 1977, p 181).

The managerial climate was also affecting social work in the 1960s. In the wake of the Seebohm Report, the introduction of social services departments and dissolution of children's departments effectively ensured that the role of chief officer within local authorities was removed from female hands. Despite their initial dominance as children's officers and their majority presence in those roles, women did not succeed in retaining a significant share of the directorships of social services departments. Of the 171 departments originally established in England and Wales, only 16 were headed by women and in a subsequent reorganisation of local government in 1974 the numbers of departments in England and Wales fell to 116, of which only 10 were headed by women. In both the Seebohm and Salmon reports the language presented changed expectations and an emphasis on managerial control and the visible outcome was certainly masculinisation at that time and subsequently (Foster 1987).

Women colluded with these changes, expecting that a greater presence of men would result in higher occupational status. Within social work, for example, Eileen Younghusband had argued particularly for a need to attract more men into the occupation, for this reason. Leaders, including women, in both occupations appear to have welcomed the changes proposed within these reports without anticipating the gendered impact. Indeed, even had they done so, it is unlikely that the women leaders would necessarily have seen this as problematic. The positions of authority had been largely confined to women who remained single in a postwar era where the supposed joys of family life were accompanied by a pitying approach to a generation of women for whom the prospect of marriage had been damaged by the deaths of a generation of men and for whom economic independence was a necessity. Presenting a career as a second-best alternative for women enabled society to ignore the possibility that the availability of opportunities for economic independence might enable women to choose not to marry. If the women themselves believed the propaganda and saw themselves as unusual compared with other women, they would be unlikely to be concerned about a greater presence of men. Indeed, a concern for the status of the occupation generally would mean that they welcomed it.

Six Steps to **Effective Management**

The last two decades have seen ongoing legislative reform of health and welfare services and an increasing emphasis on managerialism which arguably has contributed to the masculinisation of senior positions. The passage of the Sex Discrimination and Equal Pay Acts in the 1970s failed to halt the decline in the proportions of women in senior management in social services departments (Foster 1987) and by the late 1980s the absence of women was becoming a focus for criticism. In the 1990s, following the publication of the Hansard Report, the cross-party initiative Opportunity 2000 was launched in an effort to encourage large employers to appoint more women into managerial roles. The encouragement has again had an ideological emphasis on biological differences and the 'special contribution' women can make to management. Thus, much of the encouragement of women into management in the 1990s was based on revaluing 'female' qualities rather than challenging the theories of biological difference from which such stereotypes are derived.

Such an approach seeks to build on biological determinist foundations by arguing that there are 'special qualities' which women may be expected to bring into management. It is argued that these qualities result in a different style of management, a more cooperative, less confrontational, softer style which is imputed to women. Research to date has shown little evidence to support differences in leadership styles between women and men, although the arguments may be used to appeal to the rational manager concerned to maximise efficiency and utilise the skills of the workforce effectively without challenging inherently sexist assumptions. Progress made by women on these terms provides a tenuous hold on positions of power.

A choice to emphasise sex differences has marked limitations. The ways in which biological arguments have been used as a foundation for blaming women for their absence from management illustrate the dangers. The arguments used in the past have claimed that women were absent from management because they 'lacked ambition', 'lacked career commitment' and were 'too client/patient oriented'. As a result of these attributes, they were unsuited to management. These arguments underpin approaches which offer special training to women to offset their limitations and result in expectations that either require women to change to fit in to organisations which demand controlling rational managers or expect women to make a special and different contribution. There is no place for diversity amongst women.

This deficit model of women may be accompanied or replaced by explanations for their position which focus on situational barriers but the underpinning biological determinism of such explanations remains. Situational barriers arising from women's role as mothers provided a convenient rationale for the continued exclusion of women from the most senior roles. According to this explanation, women's position in the labour market is accounted for by their taking career breaks to care for their families. The argument has been based on the model of male breadwinner and female carer with women's entry into the labour market structured in ways which reinforce their responsibilities for providing physically and emotionally, rather than financially, for themselves and others. This type of explanation has resulted in initiatives to enable women to cope with the demands of their 'natural' role as mothers: childcare arrangements, flexible working, career break schemes and so forth. Many of these initiatives have been crucial in enabling women to combine responsibilities for work in the public sphere and care for family members. Although the initiatives have enabled many women, particularly middle-class white women, to progress their careers they have also perpetuated the stereotypical expectations about women's nature and priorities.

THE STRUCTURAL DIMENSIONS OF DISCRIMINATION

The main problem of biological explanations which argue that women make a 'special contribution' is that they distract attention from the power imbalance between women and men. To reveal this has been the task of feminist writers focusing on the social construction of gender relations and developing analyses of the patriarchal nature of society and presenting the sexual division of labour as a social division and changeable rather than a natural and immutable one. From this perspective the imperative to ensure greater access to management for women and members of minority ethnic groups is more a matter of social justice than economic effectiveness.

The explanations for the sexual division of labour from this perspective are rooted in the dominance of men, particularly white men, within patriarchal society and the perpetuation of the power structures to their advantage. The ideological justifications for ascribing particular characteristics to tasks is then exposed as a way of maintaining the patriarchal structure. Jobs are designated as sex related and in this designation the widespread resistance within societies to allowing women to have authority over men

Women in the caring professions

influences their access to roles within the public sphere of organisations (Alvesson & Due Billing 1997). The distribution of women and men in the workforce is the result of subtle processes of discrimination and of institutionally sexist attitudes manifested in the behaviours of women and men within organisations and of the culture these create. These ideas present a far greater strategic challenge to managers who are required to challenge stereotypes of men as well as of women if fair treatment is to be achieved.

CONCLUSION

This chapter has explored the historical dimensions of women's association with professional caring roles and some of the ideological factors which may contribute to their exclusion from management. It has sought to raise issues for the practising manager and to prompt greater consideration of gender issues. For nursing and social work, as predominantly female occupations, there is a particular challenge in managing a diverse female workforce and ensuring that the potential contribution of all can be maximised. It is a challenge to counter stereotypes about all groups but particularly about women and men. And it is an opportunity for members of both sexes to develop organisations which both challenge and change these stereotypes and to model a partnership of women and men working equitably together.

The strategies which have enabled women to combine employment and childrearing have allowed many mothers to progress careers. However, this has often required them to work a double shift and combine their responsibilities within the workplace with responsibilities for caring roles in the private sphere. There has been little indication that either social work or nursing has made significant moves to redefine traditional roles and encourage more men to enter and remain in professional caring roles or assume greater caring responsibilities in the domestic sphere. The relatively rapid movement of men through both nursing and social work into management prevents their challenging the association of caring roles with women and helps to maintain the sexual division of labour. Nor have these occupations succeeded in influencing societal attitudes towards 'caring roles' to persuade decision makers to value the tasks of carers more highly. To gain financial rewards in both occupations requires an abandonment of practitioner roles and 'progress' into management. The revaluing of caring tasks and those who undertake them lies at the heart of managing diversity.

Women are not a homogeneous group. Managing a predominantly female workforce effectively requires managers to be aware of differences amongst women and amongst men as well as to recognise similarities between women and men. The opportunities available to women and to men may have been limited by their class background or educational experiences. Their experiences will have been mediated by these factors, by their ethnic origin, their sexual orientation and their age. Their needs as employees will be affected by their life cycle, circumstances and other obligations. Although part-time work is a common feature of employment in health and social services, it is rare for opportunities to work part time to be available at senior levels and very few men work part time. According to Coyle (1995), training and development within the NHS remain ad hoc and opportunities for promotion often rely on informal networks. In such situations women continue to be disadvantaged, particularly if they are from minority ethnic groups. Enabling employees, both women and men, to maintain a balance in their commitments and ensuring that all have opportunities to develop requires managers to confront their own assumptions and to challenge those of others. Changing gendered attitudes can be beneficial to all.

References

Alvesson M, Due Billing Y 1997 Understanding gender and organizations. Sage, London

Beishon S, Virdee S, Hagell A 1995 Nursing in a multi-ethnic NHS. Policy Studies Institute, London

Carpenter M 1977 The new managerialism and professionalism in nursing. In: Stacey M, Reid M, Heath C, Dingwall R (eds) Health and the division of labour. Croom Helm, London

Carpenter, M 1978 Managerialism and the division of labour in nursing. In: Dingwall R, McIntosh J (eds) Readings in the sociology of nursing. Churchill Livingstone, Edinburgh

Coyle A 1995 Women and organisational change. Equal Opportunities Commission, Manchester

Dale J, Foster P 1986 Feminists and state welfare. Routledge and Kegan Paul, London

Dilke A, Whitley A 1894 Women's work. Methuen, London

Dingwall R, Rafferty A-M, Webster C 1988 An introduction to the social history of nursing. Routledge, London

Doyal L, Elston M E 1986 Women, health and medicine. In: Beechey V, Whitelegg E (eds) Women in Britain today. Open University Press, Milton Keynes

Women in the caring professions

Six Steps to **Effective Management**

Equal Opportunities Commission 1991 Equality management: women's employment in the NHS. Equal Opportunities Commission, Manchester

Foster J 1987 Women on the wane. Insight 2(50)

Gamarnikou E 1978 Sexual division of labour: the case of nursing. In: Kuhn A, Wolpe A-M (eds) Feminism and materialism. Routledge, London

Harrison B 1996 Not only the 'dangerous trades': women's work and health in Britain 1880–1914. Taylor and Francis, London

Kuhn A, Wolpe A-M 1978 Feminism and materialism. Routledge, London

Nottage A 1991 Women in social services: a neglected resource, HMSO, London

Report of the Committee on the Care of Children (The Curtis Report) 1946. HMSO, London

Stacey M, Reid M, Heath C, Dingwall R 1977 Heath and the division of labour. Croom Helm, London

Stibbs A (ed) 1992 Like a fish needs a bicycle. Bloomsbury, London

Ulrich B 1992 Leadership and management according to Florence Nightingale. Appleton and Lange, Norwalk

Watkin B 1975 Documents on health and social services: 1834 to the present day. Methuen, London

Wilson E 1977 Women and the welfare state. Tavistock, London

Witz A 1992 Professions and patriarchy. Routledge, London

Diversity and inequality in health care

Chapter **Four**

Researching women in primary care: the importance of the self in critical reflection

Lai Fong Chiu

- ● Introduction
- ● Involving different groups in the project
- ● Facilitating empowerment
- ● Conclusion

OVERVIEW

Action research is increasingly popular in the NHS (Myers 2000), particularly in nursing research. Although nurses are familiar with the concept of reflection, its application in action research has rarely been debated. The premise of action research is change through the participation of those who are involved in the process and an action researcher is deeply implicated in the change process as a change agent. Researchers' awareness of the self and their relationships with others in the research process is therefore crucial for the success of the project. It is particularly important to recognise, when researching among a diverse population in primary care, that researchers are often confronted with the inequalities of gender and ethnicity experienced by their participants. This chapter focuses on two personal qualities required in an action researcher that would help to facilitate participation among diverse population groups. It draws on examples from an action research project entitled

Six Steps to **Effective Management**

Woman-to-Woman: promoting cervical screening among minority ethnic women in primary care (1995–1997). The awareness of the structural inequality in social relationships and the complexity of facilitating empowerment are two important qualities for an action researcher who also wishes to become an effective change agent.

INTRODUCTION

It has already been argued in earlier chapters that our social relationships are structured by inequality. When researching women in the context of primary care, the issue of diversity and inequality takes on even greater significance since aspects of ethnicity, gender and profession will be played out. Action research, based on social change and improvement of practice, is particularly useful since it is problem focused and orientated towards both improving practice and bringing about changes in individuals and groups. This approach accords with the patient-centred and empowerment approaches currently being promoted in nursing practice.

Action research is becoming increasingly popular in the NHS (Myers 2000). Researchers embracing this method need to appreciate the importance of self-critical reflection on the research process (Meulenberg-Buskens 1996). The concept of the self helps us to see the researcher as deeply implicated in the research process. In transforming others, the researcher cannot remain untransformed. The notions of 'reflection', 'collective reflection', 'self-reflection' and 'reflective practice' have often been invoked in the literature of action research as indicators of good practice (e.g. Cornwall & Jewkes 1995, Dockery 1996, McTaggart 1997, Meulenberg-Buskens 1996, Seymour-Rolls & Hughes 1995).

The researcher's critical awareness of self and of their relationships with the participants is particularly important in carrying out action research among the diverse populations in the primary care setting. Since transformation is a goal for action research, reflective researchers need to recognise the positional power that they have in relation to the participants and to be fully aware of the effect of their own behaviours on participation. In other words, researchers need to be aware of their use of strategy, style and skills with which empowerment of participants could be enhanced.

This chapter focuses on self-awareness of the two personal aspects which are vital for successful participation in action research, using examples from an action research project, the Woman to Woman Project, which was carried out in South Yorkshire between 1995 and 1997. Its aim was to promote cervical screening to minority ethnic women in primary care.

REFLECTING ON STRUCTURAL INEQUALITY WHEN INVOLVING DIFFERENT GROUPS IN THE PROJECT

Apart from involving practice nurses from each of the six enlisted practices, the project also involved six minority groups. These were: African-Carribean (English or black English speaking); Pakistani (Mirpuri speaking); Chinese (Cantonese speaking); Bengali (Sylheti speaking); Yemeni (Arabic speaking); Vietnamese (Cantonese or Vietnamese speaking). As I reflected upon the process of involving the various groups, I recognised that power underpinned all our relationships. The decision as to which 'ethnic' groups to involve in this project was a good example of this. The funder's decision was primarily based on knowledge and assumptions that existed in the NHS in 1994. My health promotion colleague's request for the Somali group to be involved was based on her practical experience of the inequalities experienced by the Somali group in Sheffield. However, the Somali group was not defined locally or nationally as an 'ethnic' group.

Although minority groups are often sceptical of the adequacy of the OPCS categories in ethnic monitoring, ironically, these categories have the effect of legitimating the groups to which they are applied and giving them access to rights and resources that could otherwise not be claimed. For example, the Chinese, previously categorised as 'Others', were not recognised as an official category until the 1991 census. Since then, services targeted directly to the Chinese have begun to develop across the country. In contrast, the Somali group is still not recognised as a distinct minority ethnic group nationally. Without this legitimation, they are structurally powerless. The Yemenis (Arabic language group) were in a similarly weak position nationally but were recognised by the local health authority officially as a distinct and separate ethnic group within the district. As a group, they had already established a sociopolitical infrastructure, which enabled them to negotiate with agencies and authorities for resources and to deliver services to their own community. Efforts were made by local health policy makers to include them in the project.

Researching women in primary care

I was aware that by making a choice between different groups based upon the funder's brief, I was likely to perpetuate the inequality that exists among different minority groups. However, in responding to the local situation, I began to recognise that the participants and I were caught in the web of power and some decisions would ultimately have to be made under political constraints. At times, I found myself facing dilemmas that did not appear to have immediate solutions. The awareness that I had entered a set of complex social relationships that were structured by inequality helped me avoid self-laceration and to make pragmatic decisions that I believed would benefit the project and ultimately minority groups in the long run.

AWARENESS OF THE COMPLEXITY OF FACILITATING EMPOWERMENT

In the context of action research, the processes of exploring, learning and producing knowledge are underpinned by the fundamental principle of empowerment. The strategy developed to promote the cervical screening service by participants on the Woman-To-Woman Project required a close working relationship with bilingual women from minority ethnic communities. As a social group, women from the minority ethnic communities are often socially and politically marginalised and oppressed. Therefore, it was important for practitioners to recognise their own social position of power vis-à-vis the women involved (Novak 1996) and honour their rights as individuals who could identify their own health needs, make their own choices and take their own actions (Wallerstein & Bernstein 1988). This way of working requires a fundamental shift in the attitude of professionals and a critical rethinking of their role. Critical learning was introduced to practitioners during the project to enable them to become aware of the structural constraints and oppression which specific groups experience (Allman & Wallis 1996) and to develop critical consciousness and participate in the transformation of their practice (Freire 1972).

In the course of developing critical learning with participants in the project, I found myself on the one hand acting as a supportive friend providing a sympathetic ear in times of doubt and on the other as a 'researcher' systematically recording the processes either manually or by audio taping. Frequently, I had to provide the group with explanations of the principles of action research and clarify the processes needed for the project. However, I did not always explain the entire rationale for each practical step. I was aware that I was sometimes seen as the 'expert', with the corresponding social authority. In my directive mode, I found myself operating in a seemingly manipulative manner, which profoundly contradicts the ideal of empowerment and participation.

Challenges to the uncritical assumptions of practitioners regarding minority ethnic women during awareness-raising exercises caused considerable discomfort to the participants and myself. I was under considerable stress and had not made arrangements for appropriate supervision in this respect. The distraught reaction of one of the health professionals to my co-facilitator's sari (she was of mixed heritage and one of the health professionals was suspicious of her motive in dressing in a sari) also highlighted the potentially complex situational effects of the facilitators' skills and cultural identities.* Once again, I found myself caught between the conflicting roles of 'friendly facilitator' and 'agent provocateur'. This resonates with the distress facilitation as observed by Brown et al (1982) and Reason (1988).

Heron (1989) has clearly outlined the fluidity of different modes of facilitation that a facilitator can adopt in different contexts. He also suggested that our deeply held values, personal development and training affect our style. My own experiences taught me that facilitating action research requires a wide variety of skills, which must be judiciously applied. In particular, building a trust relationship is essential before challenging participants' racial or sexual attitudes, as these are extremely emotive and sensitive issues. The psychological and affective aspect of the process of transformation in action research needs to be acknowledged.

CONCLUSION

My experience supports the view that the concept of the self is important in developing critical reflection. Psychoanalysis has been regarded as an appropriate theoretical grounding for research of this nature. The Jungian concept of the wounded healer prompts us to question our own involvement in research, our cultural authority as a researcher and how our knowledge, attitudes and skills influence not only the process but also the outcomes of the

*Full details of this event can be found in Chiu L F 2000 A participatory action research study of an intercultural communication strategy for improving experience of cervical screening among minority ethnic women in the primary care setting.

Researching women in primary care

research. In the process of facilitating transformation, the researcher is deeply implicated and cannot expect to leave the research site with her 'self' untransformed. As a minority ethnic woman and a health promotion practitioner, my fellow participants and I were caught at the intersection of ethnicity, gender and professional practice. Power differentials exist between individuals and groups and these may facilitate or impede change. It is only through self-awareness that one can become a competent action researcher and an effective change agent. The understanding of the self and others is pivotal in addressing the issue of diversity in research.

Acknowledgement

The author wishes to thank all the women and health professionals who participated in the project and the NHS Cervical Screening Programme for its financial support.

References

Allman P, Wallis J 1996 Challenging the postmodern condition. In: Mayo M, Thompson J (eds) Adult learning, critical intelligence and social change. National Organisation for Adult Learning, Leicester

Brown L et al. 1982 Action research – notes on the National Seminar. In: Elliott J, Whitehead D (eds) Action-research for professional development and the improvement of schooling. Institute of Education, Cambridge

Chiu L 2000 A participatory action research study of an intercultural communication strategy for improving the experience of cervical screening among minority ethnic women in the primary care setting. Unpublished PhD thesis, University of Leeds

Cornwall A, Jewkes R 1995 What is participatory research? Social Science and Medicine 41(12):1667–1676

Dockery G 1996 Rhetoric or reality? Participatory research in the National Health Service, UK. In: De Konning K, Martin M (eds) Participatory research in health: issues and experiences. Zed Books, London

Freire P 1972 Pedagogy of the oppressed. Penguin, Harmondsworth

Heron J 1989 The facilitator's handbook. Kogan Page, London

McTaggart R (ed) 1997 Participatory action research: international contexts and consequences. State University of New York, Albany

Meulenberg-Buskens I 1996 Critical awareness in participatory research: an approach towards teaching and learning. In: De Konning K, Martin M (eds) Participatory research in health: issues and experiences. Zed Books, London

Myers J 2000 Qualitative methods in health-related action research. In: Pope C, Mays N (eds) Qualitative research in health care. BMJ Books, London

Diversity and inequality in health care

Novak T 1996 Empowerment and the politics of poverty. In: Humphries B (ed) Critical perspectives on empowerment. Venture Press, Birmingham

Reason P 1988 Developments in methodology. In: Reason P (ed) Human inquiry in action: developments in new paradigm research. Sage, London

Seymour-Rolls S, Hughes I 1995 Participatory action research: getting the job done. Action Research Electronic Reader. Action Research On the Web. I.Hughes@cchs.usyd.edu.au

Wallerstein N, Bernstein E 1988 Empowerment education: Freire's ideas adapted to health education. Health Education Quarterly 15(4):379–394

Researching women in primary care

THE ETHICAL AND LEGAL FRAMEWORK

Chapter **Five**

Equality, justice and tolerance: ethical foundations for the management of diversity

Martin Johnston

OVERVIEW

Management entails control and necessarily establishes an imbalanced power relationship, where an individual or group is able to exert authority over others. The essence of the power relationship is that management decisions have consequences for those who are managed, whether they be other employees of an institution or service users. There is nothing inherently unethical about this but failure to recognise the one-sided nature of the power relationship can lead to a failure to exercise responsibility appropriately. The exercise of power without responsibility is inherently unethical.

The primary concern of this chapter is an exploration of some key concepts and themes in ethics which have much to offer in terms of providing a secure foundation for the appropriate exercise of power. In a departure from fairly standard treatments of ethics in nursing, the main focus will not be on competing broad ethical theories like deontological and utilitarian approaches but rather on three key concepts: equality, justice and tolerance. Close examination of these concepts should go some way towards establishing an appropriate foundation from which practitioners can identify and develop for themselves a framework for practice in what will no doubt remain a highly contentious area.

> **Objectives**
>
> This chapter explores the following themes and issues:
> - equality and its origins
> - justice as fairness and its application in the nursing context
> - tolerance: its scope and limitations.

EQUALITY

In what is at first sight a fairly clear statement, the UKCC makes an explicit commitment to the principle of equality among persons. Item 7 of the *Code of professional conduct* reads as follows.

> Recognise and respect the uniqueness and dignity of each patient and client, and respond to their need for care, irrespective of their ethnic origin, religious beliefs, personal attributes, the nature of their health problems or any other factor. (UKCC 1992)

Though such a claim may strike us as laudable, as soon as we try to move from rhetoric to practice a number of difficulties are encountered. The primary source of these stems from something essentially paradoxical in the formulation. There is an implicit acknowledgement of difference in the UKCC's statement and in dealing with diversity this book shares that acknowledgement, which initially clashes with any kind of absolute conception of equality. Add to this the influence on nursing theory of humanist writers like Rogers (1989) and the current emphasis on patient/client autonomy in ethical literature (Beauchamp & Childress 1989, Madder 1997, Tschudin 1990) and we have apparently conflicting principles which advocate a standardised egalitarian approach to health care provision whilst at the same time entreating practitioners to recognise and value the unique nature of individuals. In exploring this paradox, we may not arrive at definitive conclusions but a more careful analysis of the concept of equality may help to illuminate the nature of the difficulties.

Equality as a property of things

The basic question to be addressed in this section is 'What do we mean when we describe things as equal?'. In dealing with this question we shall begin with the more mundane aspects of equality generally before moving on to the more interesting aspects of the idea of equality among persons.

The origins of the idea of equality

In a formal sense we may derive the idea of equality from arithmetic. In this sense the concept of equality comes to be synonymous with 'is identical to'; hence 2+3 equals (is identical to) 5. But whilst this may get us somewhere in terms of abstract objects like numbers, it does little to inform our concepts of equality between material things. In attempting to establish a broad idealism, which need not concern our purposes, Plato (1987a) presents the following difficulty.

> 'Here is a further step,' said Socrates. 'We admit, I suppose, that there is such a thing as equality – not the equality of stick to stick and stone to stone, and so on, but something beyond all that and distinct from it – absolute equality. Are we to admit this or not?
> 'Yes indeed,' said Simmias, 'most emphatically.'
> 'And do we know what it is?'
> 'Certainly.'
> 'Where did we get our knowledge? Was it not from the particular examples we mentioned just now? Was it not from seeing equal sticks or stones or other equal objects that we got the notion of equality, although it is something quite distinct from them? Look at it in this way. Is it not true that equal stones and sticks sometimes, without changing in themselves, appear equal to one person and unequal to another?'
> 'Certainly.'
> 'Well now, have you ever thought that things which were absolutely equal were unequal or that equality was inequality?'
> 'No, never, Socrates.'
> 'Then these equal things are not the same as absolute equality.'
> 'Not in the least, as I see it, Socrates.' (pp 122–123)

Plato's intentions here go far beyond our area of interest but a key feature is identified in the quoted passage. It concerns a move away from a formal account of equality – like the arithmetical conception – to a more practical everyday account. The idea of 'absolute equality' is too restrictive. Instead of thinking of equality as 'is identical

Ethical foundations for the management of diversity

to', we move to a broader account of equality as 'is the same as'. In this sense two ties, two cars or Plato's sticks and stones may be equal without being identical in a strictly formal sense; what we mean in describing such objects as equal is that they are the same. But an important additional element creeps in here, particularly when we talk of manufactured objects like cars. This element can be described in terms of purposes. Two cars may be equal in terms of getting their owners from A to B; in this sense, a Porsche is equal to a Reliant Robin. But clearly that is not the whole story. If an individual is more image conscious or keen to show off his or her wealth then the equivalence between the two makes of car, in terms of providing a means of transportation, is no longer the issue.

In making matters practical, then, the picture has become more complicated. We now have a notion of equality as being synonymous with 'is the same as', but this raises the additional question of 'Is the same as in what respect?'. And it is this question which is central in a discussion of equality among persons.

Equality among persons

Plato's (1987b) account in *The republic* is, strictly speaking, more an account of inequality among persons. For him there exist significant differences between groups of individuals which merit different treatment in society. His view of the necessary subordination of women and acceptance of slavery make his account rightly unpalatable to many modern readers. Nevertheless, even now there are still those who advocate meritocracy and divisions along functional lines as being an inherently good thing. Indeed, the modern health service is just such an organisation; hierarchical systems reward those at the top more than those at the bottom and such situations are often seen as basic 'facts of life'. For many, then, though the individuals and groups may have become more expansive, the divisions remain. In addressing our earlier question, the respect in which persons are equal in these terms is defined functionally.

To explore such matters further we must part company with Plato and go on to consider the work of Jean-Jacques Rousseau.

Rousseau's account

Rousseau may be accused of many things – a certain historical and anthropological naiveté, a penchant for romanticism in his view of human nature – but a more impassioned and heartfelt plea for equality among persons is hard to find. By way of example, consider the following.

> The first man who, having enclosed a piece of land, thought of saying 'This is mine' and found people simple enough to believe him, was the true founder of civil society. How many crimes, wars, murders; how much misery and horror the human race would have been spared if someone had pulled up the stakes and filled in the ditch and cried out to his fellow men: 'Beware of listening to this impostor. You are lost if you forget that the fruits of the earth belong to everyone and that the earth itself belongs to no one!' (Rousseau 1984a, p 109)

The essential theme in Rousseau's work is that 'civilisation' involves a departure from the state of nature in which human beings are created equal. In these terms the cost of membership of society is high, since it is through organisation and the division of labour that inequalities emerge. Notice the sharp contrast with Plato's view; inequalities are the product of human activity and as such fit the contemporary accounts where writers talk of the social construction of inequality.

And yet there is a sense in which none of this is inevitable. It may well be the case that we cannot reverse the course of human history and return to the state of nature – a state which is representative of Rousseau's romanticism – but that is not to say that we must accept the status quo and the actual inequalities which do exist. The whole idea of the social contract (Rousseau 1984b) concerns ways in which individuals can obtain the advantages associated with life in communities without sacrificing their individuality. But the key issue concerns who is involved in the drafting and subsequent signing of the contract. Or, put another way, which inequalities are we prepared to tolerate and who should be involved in reaching that decision?

Equality in nursing

Our brief historical sojourn has provided us with examples of accounts of the nature of equality in both a formal and applied sense. In the applied sense, the most important distinction is between those views which take a basic equality among persons as given and those which take the view that there are marked differences at birth, which subsequently come to substantiate differential treatment in terms of one's place in society. In many respects what we have is a version of the standard 'nature versus nurture' debate but deciding which side of the debate to favour is of crucial importance for nurses and particularly for those nurses whose decisions have marked consequences for large numbers of people.

We are now in a position to return to item 7 of the UKCC's *Code of professional conduct*. In terms of our previous discussion, then, we can identify something of a compromise in the UKCC's position. On the one hand, there is a recognition of differences between individuals on the basis of such factors as religious belief, ethnic group and so on but this is coupled with the view that such differences should have no influence on the provision of nursing care. Recognition of difference and diversity, then, is not in itself a bad thing; indeed, it is necessarily entailed in the view that each individual is unique. What matters, however, is our response to such differences.

The essence of the UKCC's position here seems to be that with respect to the provision of nursing care, all individuals are equal in something like an absolute sense. But it is one thing to voice support for a universal principle of equality, quite another to act consistently on the basis of such an assertion. Essentially we are talking about operationalising a general ethical ideal which in the context of our present discussion can be viewed as an issue concerning the distribution of resources. This brings us to our second theme – justice.

JUSTICE

For our purposes it is the idea of distributive justice which is most important. If equality among persons is to make sense then one way to measure whether or not it is applied in concrete terms is to consider how resources are allocated. We have already noted that resource allocation decisions have to be made, so the concern is not with the making of decisions in themselves – these are a feature of contemporary health care provision – but rather with the foundations upon which such decisions are made. But just as equality proved to be a complex notion once subjected to closer analysis, so too is justice. The essential core of the idea revolves around deciding who deserves what. So we shall begin our discussion by considering a number of options which suggest ways in which distribution should be organised.

Making matters material

Beauchamp & Childress (1989) identify six possible material principles of justice.

1. To each an equal share.
2. To each according to need.
3. To each according to merit.
4. To each according to status.
5. To each according to effort.
6. To each according to free market exchanges. (p 261)

Each of these principles is best viewed as a mechanism for the distribution of resources and for our purposes, that resource is health care. In spite of this commonalty, it is immediately apparent that some, if not all, of these principles are mutually incompatible and yet all have been proposed at some time or another by their adherents as the best encapsulation of the nature of justice. But this offers little by way of practical information for difficult decision making. Which, if any, of these formulations are we to accept and employ? It is no help to point to their illustrious supporters, since even the illustrious are prone to error from time to time. Nor does it help matters to consider that each of these formulations has been used in support of actual resource allocation decisions at some time or another. What we need is to explore the issue further and it is here that the work of John Rawls (1991) provides a number of valuable insights.

Justice as fairness

Rawls' prime concern is not with which of the material principles of justice should be adopted by any given community but rather with the manner in which such a decision is made. His famous description of the veil of ignorance leads some to doubt the practical applicability of his account to actual decision making but this is to make a quite fundamental mistake. There is a sense in which distinguishing the theoretical and applied aspects of Rawls' work is artificial but so long as it is borne in mind that this is only in the interests of clarity for illustrative purposes then, as a strategy, it has some value. We begin, then, with the theoretical position.

The theoretical position

Rawls' veil of ignorance establishes a set of conditions under which the material principles of justice for a given community are to be established. In this position participants have no knowledge of their particular talents, needs or preferences but are endowed with an instrumental rationality. The idea is that decisions reached under such conditions are free from bias and are those to which all would subscribe. This establishes an important difference between behaviour which is dictated by a rule and behaviour which is genuinely rule governed, where those following the rule have a vested and personal interest in its application. From this Rawls argues that we can establish two primary principles of justice.

> First: each person is to have an equal right to the most extensive basic liberty compatible with a similar liberty for others. Second: social and economic inequalities are to be arranged so that they are both (a) reasonably expected to be to everyone's advantage, and (b) attached to positions and offices open to all. (Rawls 1991, p 60)

But Rawls' position has often been criticised for its idealism, in the sense that it is hard to imagine the detail of the original position ever being achievable for a given human community. Nonetheless, even if we reject his conclusions concerning actual principles of justice, we can still make use of his work in practical settings.

Practical issues

The most important lesson, for our purposes, to be drawn from Rawls' work is the manner in which decisions are reached. True, creating the original position in practice is impossible but we can move towards approximations of it. The key issue is participation and representation in the decision-making process. The actual constraints of general management may present barriers to this but nonetheless developments towards interdisciplinary practice and education represent an attempt to progress towards the ideal. We are dealing here with the basic foundations of liberal democracy. It is not necessary that every individual affected be involved in decision making, but it is necessary that their interests are represented. Clearly the involvement of service users is a vital component in all of this.

Justice and nurse management

Our next step is to develop these ideas within a nursing context. There are two main issues here. First, can we apply Rawls' derived principles to nursing and second, what can be learned from his general method?

Applying the principles

It would be a mistake to think that Rawls provides us with some kind of ethical panacea to solve all problems associated with distributive justice. In fact, he argues that in talking of the first principles of justice he is referring to a broad sociopolitical level which concerns the ways in which a society's institutions are set up and run. (Institutions here being conceived widely, to include government agencies, courts, marriage and the like.) In this sense it is not an individual morality, though any subsequent development of individual moral principles must not conflict with the first principles of justice.

The difficulty in applying this to a nursing context is that we appear to be somewhere in the middle. Nursing ethics are not just based on individual principles, but then neither do they operate solely at the broader sociopolitical level. In the United Kingdom the NHS remains a major government agency and is influenced by political decision making, but in terms of day-to-day practice nurses confront difficult decisions very much as individuals. The fundamental problem here is identifying those areas of practice over which a nurse has genuine control, since it makes no sense to find fault with an individual's behaviour if they could not have done otherwise (Aristotle 1991).

The nursing context

The central notion here is accountability. To whom is a nurse accountable? At the most basic level the answer is perfectly clear: a nurse is accountable to his or her patients. But then we must also take into account responsibilities towards the profession's governing body and employers. And indeed, such additional responsibilities, particularly towards employers, become all the more acute the higher up the chain of management a nurse rises. As a rough rule of thumb we could say that the greater the power (power being here measured in terms of the numbers of individuals affected by a decision) a nurse is able to exercise then the greater is the range of their corresponding responsibility. But the confounding variable here concerns the extent to which a nurse has any genuine control over broader policy decisions. Nurses are often in the difficult position of having to respond to policies implemented at a higher level over which they have little or no control, which inevitably creates a tension. And the nurse manager is more likely to be in such a position, depending upon the nature of the particular practices which a hospital board has with regard to policy formation.

Some illustrations

Suppose we have a situation in a particular hospital where the policy is that smokers who refuse to attempt to give up smoking are denied access to types of treatment which are rendered ineffective if the patient continues to smoke. Present such a scenario to any group of individuals and a diversity of opinion is likely to emerge. There will be those who wholeheartedly endorse the policy, those who endorse it with qualifications (for example, only if others whose lifestyle choices render them vulnerable to disease and injury – like those who participate in dangerous sport, those who pay no attention to diet, those who take no exercise and the like – are similarly treated) and those who vehemently oppose it. Now we do not have to decide here who is right; rather, we are concerned with the conditions which give rise to the implementation of such a policy. It is a relatively easy thing to impose such a policy, it is another matter to establish genuine support for it. Essentially this is the difference between following a rule and being governed by it outlined above. And it is here that the lessons from Rawls have a direct application. The key issue is how such a policy is established and by whom. Participation and consultation are the necessary prerequisites if we are to be anything more than slavish rule followers.

Or take the fairly common practice of setting age limits on candidates for organ transplant. Again, the issue is one where implementation is a relatively straightforward matter but where the perceived fairness of any particular policy is open to question. Decisions like these are uncomfortable and it is easy to criticise those who make them when they run contrary to our own hopes and aspirations but nonetheless they have to be made. Again, the key issues appear to be participation, consultation and representation.

Taking a different type of example, consider the practice of triage in busy A&E units. The whole point of triage is to establish priorities for treatment in terms of medical need, the most urgent cases being treated first. In this example we have quite a clear case where any absolute notion of equality is abandoned and rightly so. Indeed, it is just this type of scenario which illustrates the second of Rawls' principles. But it is not the case that representation and consultation are unimportant here; rather, it is reasonable to assume that most people would endorse the view that those most seriously ill be treated first and so their compliance with such a procedure may be assumed. Of course, there may be actual instances where individuals object to this procedure but our first response in such matters is to direct attention to the benefits of such an approach to the individual concerned, if he or she were in such a life-threatening situation. Though not strictly speaking Rawlsian, part of the appeal here is to get the individual to see the situation from a less directly self-interested position, in spite of using self-interest as a starting point.

Interim conclusions

What has emerged, then, from our discussion of justice so far is the importance of the manner in which decisions regarding the allocation of resources are made. Individual nurses and groups of nurses will have varying degrees of control of these procedures but clearly the greater the level of control they have, the greater is their level of accountability for those decisions. In this section we have explored some of the issues which require consideration and central among these is the requirement that those affected by decisions be involved either directly or through some form of appropriate representation. This leaves us with our third major theme for consideration – tolerance.

TOLERANCE

Whereas the previous section dealt with issues which can be described as the broad policy level, this section will consider matters at a more day-to-day practical level. We can have the most just policies and procedures imaginable in place but these will mean nothing if those who have to effectively implement them pay no attention to the subtleties of that implementation in the specific context. No policy can account for every possible scenario, hence it is vital that we consider additional elements of importance, central to which is the idea of tolerance.

Foundations of tolerance

We can identify at least two senses in which the word, 'tolerance' is used, of value to our present purposes. Both, however, share a common foundation in terms of entreating us to put up with or permit actions, opinions or ideas of which we disapprove. In an everyday sense this can be interpreted as a kind of non-interference in the preferences of others and this sense is very much in evidence in item 7 of the UKCC's *Code of professional conduct*. I personally may not wish to be a practising Christian (or adherent of any other religious creed) but I should be tolerant of others' wishes to be so. This much is largely uncontentious in the liberal democracies. And the same is taken to be true (if not more so) of attitudes towards other aspects of individuals over which they have no control, such as their ethnic group. But, strictly speaking, these types of attitudes do not amount to tolerance. Smith (1997) sets the scene for an account of tolerance as follows:

> 'To tolerate is to allow behaviour of which one disapproves. Two elements are vital. First, tolerance requires tension between the activity permitted and the person doing the tolerating. I cannot tolerate what I do not disapprove of. Second, in order to tolerate some activity, a person must have a moral standing to disallow that activity. I cannot tolerate what it is not my prerogative to not tolerate. (pp 32–33)

Now the second of these elements clearly deals with aspects like a person's ethnic group; it is clearly absurd to suggest that someone has the right or prerogative to object to another's ethnic group. Certainly, there may be those who in private adhere to racist dogma whilst publicly acting in accordance with, say, equal opportunities policy but let us be clear that this does not amount to tolerance. But it is those other aspects of an individual's behaviour which are freely chosen which become the proper object of inquiry. And here we return to Smith's first element, the foundations of disapproval.

Broadly consistent with Smith's view, Almond (1997) warns against taking the view that tolerance is somehow equivalent to moral neutrality. In many respects tolerance has to be viewed as the setting aside or suspension of usual moral requirements and consequently requires further justification. Viewed in this way, Smith (1997) rightly proceeds to explore whether tolerance is in fact a good thing. This is not our concern here but it is important to distinguish the two senses of tolerance at work in what follows. For the sake of brevity, we shall refer to them as the everyday sense and the technical sense.

Making matters practical

If we return to the example given on p 106, the differences between these two senses should become clear. In the example of the policy towards smokers where treatment is refused, part of any objection to it involves the everyday sense of tolerance. Human beings generally are prone to error and often make mistakes in their choices, some of which may have quite disastrous consequences for their health, so it is nothing short of intolerance to subsequently punish them for their mistakes. And clearly there is something in this view. But in the current climate of health care delivery where resources are finite, resource allocation decisions have a very real impact. Treating one individual may implicitly involve not treating someone else even though the second individual may not be immediately identifiable. In this way we may wish to question the virtue of tolerating (technical sense) the smokers' refusal to attempt to give up the habit. As before, it is not within our current remit to settle the matter one way or another; rather, it is to notice the complexity of the issue and identify pertinent facets of the argument.

Limits on tolerance

What emerges from examples like the one above is that we should give due consideration to the possibility of limits on tolerance. But for this view to be viable, we must then argue the case for any such limits which we may wish to impose. This general approach may run contrary to the standard historical ethos of professions like nursing and medicine, where need is often seen as the only quali-fying condition for the receipt of care, but is arguably the reality of contemporary provision. Jiwa (1996) illustrates the kind of diffi-culty encountered when dealing with the demanding patient prone to acts of self-harm whilst under the influence of alcohol, who subsequently refuses treatment offered, in terms of time wasted on the part of professionals. Although he stops short of delineating precise conditions when treatment or attendance may be refused, nonetheless Jiwa makes the issue very clear: is it fair that one unco-operative individual should be able to make 'excessive' demands upon the time of health care professionals?

Approaching matters from the opposite end, Orr & Genesen (1997) attempt to argue the case for giving special consideration to requests for 'inappropriate' treatment on the grounds of religious belief. Their case generally requires that we recognise the impor-tance of religious belief in a person's whole life view and conse-quently continue to provide treatment even where there are good medical reasons to consider this futile. And indeed, numerous agencies already recognise the importance of religious belief and the need to respect the views of others even when these are not shared by practitioners, all of which is consistent with the everyday sense of tolerance. (It is doubtful that the technical sense applies here, since another's religious beliefs are arguably not something which I have a right to object to.)

These two examples highlight the difficulties associated with any decision not to offer care and Lowe et al (1995) point to the very real danger of introducing prejudice into decision making under the guise of technical jargon and apparently rational decision-making procedures, but this does not of itself make the issue go away. If anything, it places a greater responsibility upon decision makers to confront the value basis of their decisions and argue for them or revise them accordingly.

CONCLUSION

As is fairly common with a chapter such as this, the reader may well be left with a sense that more questions have been raised than have been answered but it would be a mistake to presume that this is a bad thing. The broad territory is such that we should be suspicious of quick-fix solutions and easy systems for problem solving. And indeed, it would go entirely against the tone of arguments presented, with their concern for participation and consultation, to suggest any definitive answers to the problems raised by dealing with diversity. At most, what has been delivered is a starting point from which potential answers may be explored but it is in the actual context of situations dealt with that the answers will ultimately be found. It is often considered unfashionable to take a moral point of view and the temptation for professionals is to avoid dealing with value judgements. But value judgements are an integral part of nursing care so rather than avoid them, the task is to confront them head on for what they are and establish them on as secure foundations as we are able.

References

Almond B 1997 Counselling for tolerance. Journal of Applied Philosophy 14(1):19–30

Aristotle 1991 The Nicomachean ethics. Oxford University Press, Oxford

Beauchamp T L, Childress J F 1989 Principles of biomedical ethics. Oxford University Press, Oxford

Jiwa M 1996 Autonomy: the need for limits. Journal of Medical Ethics 22(6):340–343

Lowe M, Kerridge I H, Mitchell K R 1995 'These sorts of people don't do very well': race and allocation of health care resources. Journal of Medical Ethics 21(6): 356–360

Madder H 1997 Existential autonomy: why patients should make their own choices. Journal of Medical Ethics 23(4):221–225

Orr R D, Genesen L B 1997 Requests for 'inappropriate' treatment based on religious beliefs. Journal of Medical Ethics 23(3):142–147

Plato 1987a Phaedo. In: The last days of Socrates. Penguin, London

Plato 1987b The republic. Penguin, London

Rawls J 1991 A theory of justice. Oxford University Press, Oxford

Rogers C 1989 On becoming a person: a therapist's view of psychotherapy. Constable, London

Rousseau J-J 1984a A discourse on inequality. Penguin, London

Rousseau J-J 1984b Of the social contract: or principles of political right. Harper and Row, London

Smith T 1997 Tolerance and forgiveness: virtues or vices? Journal of Applied Philosophy 14(1):31–41

Tschudin V 1990 Ethics in nursing: the caring relationship. Heinemann Nursing, London

United Kingdom Central Council 1992 Code of professional conduct. UKCC, London

Ethical foundations for the management of diversity

Application **5:1**

Martin Johnston

Equality, justice and tolerance: from rhetoric to practice

INTRODUCTION

Ahmad (1990) provides a useful case to illustrate a number of the points raised in the preceding chapter. The case of the Commission for Racial Equality *v* David Roper was based upon the defendant's refusal to allow entry to his premises to a black student midwife, being seen as a breach of the Race Relations Act 1976. Ahmad quotes the presiding judge as follows:

> The point was made on behalf of the defendant that every man has his right to refuse admittance to people in his home, but where you were taking on the advantages and benefits of the Health Service and the facilities provided for medical care and treatment you cannot in our view, where you have made an appointment for medical people to come to your home to see your wife, allow one in because they are white and refuse admittance to the other because they are of non-British racial origin. It would be a sad state for this country if that were the case. (Ahmad 1990, p 52)

In so ruling, the judge found Roper to be in breach of Section 31 of the Race Relations Act 1976. But our concern is not with the legal ruling; rather we wish to consider the ethical basis of the decision in relation to the three key concepts of equality, justice and tolerance.

EQUALITY

In this context we have something like an absolute conception of equality. The key issue is that with respect to the provision of care the only important characteristic is professional status. Qualities such as ethnic group and religious persuasion are viewed as irrelevant in terms of providing a basis for judging professional competence. In

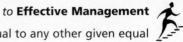
this respect, one health professional is equal to any other given equal levels of qualification.

JUSTICE

The case nicely illustrates the idea of the contractual approach to justice. Essentially the issue is this. If I reap the benefits of some communal service then I must correspondingly limit the more radical aspects of my liberty. In the ruling it is taken that one generally has the right to refuse entry to one's property but that this right is waived when one enters into some kind of contract with a public agency from which one gains some kind of benefit. People may have the right to prejudiced beliefs in their own home but they do not have the right to inflict these beliefs on others, particularly where those others are offering a substantive gain to the individual as part of statutory service provision.

TOLERANCE

The technical sense of tolerance in relation to this type of case has already been dealt with in the preceding chapter, so it is with the everyday sense that we are concerned here. Quite clearly, the ruling identifies a very definite limit on tolerance. In this case the defendant's views are considered to be essentially wrong and consequently not worthy of respect. Whatever an individual's negative beliefs concerning the importance of the ethnic origin of health care professionals, they do not deserve to be tolerated.

CONCLUSION

Though much of what has been discussed depends upon an interpretation of the judge's ruling, nonetheless the example begins to tease out some of the complexities of applying the three key concepts. Of course, there is still room for debate as to whether this is all ultimately justifiable but the quest for such justification presumably lies somewhere in the direction described.

References

Ahmad A 1990 Practice with care. Race Equality Unit Personal Social
    Services, London

From rhetoric to practice

113

Application 5:2

Carol Baxter, Ann Gallagher

Blowing the whistle on racism in services: ethical, professional and legal aspects

INTRODUCTION

Over the last 15 years, a number of professionals in health and social care achieved fame and, in some quarters, notoriety by going public about practices they considered unethical, unprofessional and illegal. In 1989 Dr Chris Chapman, a senior scientist at Leeds General Infirmary, went public about scientific fraud (Hugill 1992). In 1990 charge nurse Graham Pink shared his concerns about standards of care for elderly patients at Stepping Hill Hospital in *The Guardian* newspaper (Brindle 1990). In that same year, Dr Helen Zeitlin spoke out about shortages of nurses at Bromsgrove (Snell 1992). Dr Stephen Bolsin shared his concerns about high mortality rates in children undergoing heart surgery at Bristol (*Guardian* 1998). His testimony led to a television documentary in 1996.

Reports of negligence and abuse have been abundant in health care in recent years. It seems that at least on a weekly basis, the public is informed about harm (physical and psychological) to individuals or groups caused by the misconduct of individuals and the failure of institutions. Many of these harms came to light as a result of an individual speaking out, usually at great personal cost.

Whistle blowing has been defined as 'the act of calling to public attention abuses or dangers which jeopardise public safety and which would not otherwise be publicised' (Chadwick & Tadd 1992). James (in Callahan 1988) goes on to make a helpful distinction between internal and external whistle blowing. *Internal* whistle blowing occurs when an employee discloses wrongdoing to higher management within the organisation, going over the heads of immediate managers. *External* whistle blowing occurs when the employee makes the disclosure to those outside the organisation, to the media, public interest groups or regulatory bodies, for example. In 1995, Hunt wrote that:

> Whistleblowing surfaced in the UK health service in an atmosphere of apprehension and anxiety. Economic recession and public expenditure cuts, combined with the imposition of commercial-style management on the National Health Service, have threatened standards of care, disempowered health care professionals and almost certainly created new conditions for negligence and abuse, and new opportunities for fraud and corruption. (p xv)

Two developments in the late 1990s offered hope for a change in culture regarding whistle blowing: the introduction of clinical governance and changes in the law which resulted in the Public Interest Disclosure Act 1998.

There have been many media reports about racial abuse and harassment in health care but few have appeared under the umbrella of whistle blowing. An exception is the case of the black health visitor Desmond Smith, who was a victim of racial discrimination and who was awarded record damages from Hounslow and Spelthorne Health Authority (Health Visitor 1993, p 114, Hunt 1995, p xix). Mr Smith was 'racially abused by a client in the presence of colleagues' (Baddeley 1993). Reporting the incident did not lead to an investigation. Instead, the health authority investigated a later complaint against Mr Smith by the client. Mr Smith was suspended for 'breaching confidentiality' after sending a disciplinary hearing dossier to his MP. The MP had returned the dossier to Mr Smith's manager. He subsequently contacted Freedom to Care, a non-profit-making company which supports employees who speak out about issues of public concern, which directed him to individuals and organisations which would help him. Mr Smith was exonerated and awarded £27 000. The manager in this case was criticised for continuing to make allegations against Mr Smith which had been withdrawn in an industrial tribunal (Baddeley 1993).

Managers in nursing have a number of key roles to play in relation to whistle blowing and racism. They have a *primary role* in working towards the development of a positive care and work environment where diversity is valued and individuals are treated with respect and benefited rather than harmed by encounters with staff and colleagues. The dictum 'lead by example' is also pertinent here. Managers have a *secondary role* in ensuring that where concerns about racial harassment or abuse are expressed, they are taken seriously, investigated thoroughly and responded to appropriately. Managers may have to report the concerns of others and/or their own concerns to senior management, professional bodies or legal authorities. The nurse manager, having exhausted the usual reporting mechanism, may feel compelled to 'whistle blow'. Managers also have a *tertiary role* in developing strategies, policies

Blowing the whistle on racism in services

or protocols which provide an effective and supportive mechanism for staff to express concerns about the environment of care and work. These strategies should have a sound ethical, professional and legal basis.

The remainder of this chapter focuses on a case outline which raises key issues for managers in relation to race and whistle blowing. The case appeared in the *Asian Times and Caribbean Times* (Enisuoh 1999).

Case study 5.2.1   Chandra

Chandra worked with a support team which was supposed to care for young people with learning difficulties. She enjoyed her work and found it fulfilling. She was, however, concerned that some white members of staff were making racist comments about black and Asian service users. Despite challenging the workers concerned, the racism continued. Eventually, Chandra was forced to do something that she was reluctant to do: she blew the whistle to management. 'I couldn't believe that it was going on,' she says.

'I'm Asian and they felt nothing about making racist comments in front of me. What was worse was how they treated vulnerable people in their care.'

While her line manager did superficially try to take action (he called a staff meeting to discuss the issues and organised a race awareness training session) the situation didn't change. All but two of the staff boycotted the race awareness training session and most continued to make racist comments. Meanwhile, Chandra was ostracised by the rest of the staff for 'telling tales' to management.

For months, she faced hostility from her co-workers. Frustrated, Chandra went back to her manager, who seemed irritated that she was still pursuing the issue and fobbed her off. Disappointed with the lack of support from her co-workers and manager, Chandra decided to succumb and resigned from her job. (From Enisuoh 1999)

It is not clear from the case outline to what level of management Chandra reported her initial concerns. However, the case does raise the following issues regarding the appropriate action of nurses and managers when concerns about racism in practice are voiced.

- Ethical and professional rationale for action when concerns are raised about racial harassment or abuse in a care and work environment.
- Management responses when concerns are raised.
- Legal recourse for whistle blowers.

Ethical and legal framework

ETHICAL AND PROFESSIONAL RATIONALE FOR ACTION

Ethics permeates all aspects of professional practice. The concern of ethics can be said to be with right conduct and good character; that is, doing the right thing and displaying morally desirable character traits. Although there is no consensus on ethical approaches to be adopted in health care, there is an ever-growing body of knowledge. Some practitioners may look to codes of conduct for rules of thumb to guide their actions. If managers are registered nurses, they may look to the UKCC *Code of professional conduct* (1992) and other UKCC documents for guidelines regarding their actions in relation to patients/clients and staff.

Codes have various functions but a fundamental function is that they express the ethical obligations of the profession. It can be argued that the UKCC Code outlines Chandra's (if she is a registered nurse) and the nurse manager's obligations to ensure that patients are benefited by health care, to ensure that no harm comes to patients/clients (or indeed staff), to ensure that patients/clients make informed choices and to treat patients/clients fairly and with respect. A number of clauses are particularly relevant.

Clause 1

> Act always in such a manner as to promote and safeguard the interests and well-being of patients and clients.

If staff are making racist comments towards clients, already a vulnerable group due to their learning difficulty, their interests are unlikely to be promoted and their (psychological) well-being is jeopardised.

Clause 7

> Recognise and respect the uniqueness and dignity of each patient and client, and respond to their need for care, irrespective of their ethnic origin, religious beliefs, personal attributes, the nature of their health problem or any other factor.

As the case is reported, it seems clear that the uniqueness and dignity of each patient and client are *not* being recognised and respected. They are being discriminated against on the basis of race. In addition to considering the actions of individuals in this case, a conscientious and reflective manager should also consider institutional aspects of racism. In the recent inquiry into the death of Stephen Lawrence, a definition of racism in general terms was provided; it 'consists of conduct or words or practices which

Blowing the whistle on racism in services

disadvantage or advantage people because of their colour, culture or ethnic origin. In its more subtle form it is as damaging as in its overt form' (MacPherson 1999, p 19). Institutional racism is notoriously difficult to define and this is acknowledged.

Three other clauses of the UKCC *Code of professional conduct* are relevant to Chandra's case.

11. Report to an appropriate person or authority, having regard to the physical, psychological and social effects on patients and clients, any circumstances in the environment of care which could jeopardise standards of practice.
12. Report to an appropriate person or authority any circumstances in which safe and appropriate care for patients and clients cannot be provided.
13. Report to an appropriate person or authority where it appears that the health and safety of colleagues is at risk, as such circumstances may compromise standards of practice and care;

In the UKCC's *Guidelines for professional practice* (1996, p 21) it is pointed out that nurses:

...may be afraid to speak out for fear of losing your job. However, if you do not report your concerns, you may be in breach of the Code of Professional Conduct. You may also have concerns over inappropriate behaviour by a colleague and feel it necessary to make your concerns known. You will need to report your concerns to the appropriate person or authority, depending on the type of concerns. You may find it necessary to discuss these decisions with other colleague or a membership organisation.

The obligation of managers registered with the UKCC is to 'assess the report and communicate it to senior managers where appropriate' (UKCC 1996, p 22). In this case it is clear that the health and welfare of clients *and* staff are compromised. Chandra was ostracised and eventually left her position. Geoff Hunt, an authority on whistle blowing, is quoted as saying 'We now have plenty of evidence that whistle blowing affects health. When people are put under that kind of stress in highly charged atmospheres it can cause all kinds of illness' (Dobson 1998). Given that the above clauses have been violated in this case, it is clear that there is an ethical and professional imperative for action.

MANAGEMENT RESPONSES WHEN CONCERNS ARE RAISED

The case study states that 'while her (Chandra's) line manager did superficially try to take action (he called a staff meeting to discuss the issue and organised a race awareness training session) the situation didn't change'. When Chandra returned to her manager with her concerns he 'seemed irritated that she was still pursuing the issue and fobbed her off'. As indicated above, managers are obligated to ensure that the welfare and well-being of patients/clients and staff are not jeopardised. This manager may well have taken the view that there was nothing more he could do; however, racist behaviour continued. Chandra had the choice of taking her concerns higher or leaving the service. She chose the latter. The problem identified by Chandra focuses on the behaviour of individual staff members who clearly have negative attitudes towards those from other ethnic groups. Attitudes are difficult to change and it may be that if the attitudes and behaviour of these staff members cannot be changed, then disciplinary action is a necessary managerial response. Managers in these situations may feel torn between their obligations to colleagues and their obligations to clients/patients. In this case, of course, both staff (Chandra) and clients require protection. Staff who work in health care must understand who they are there for. As stated above, managers have a number of roles in eliminating the need for whistle blowing and in ensuring that where staff wish to raise concerns there is a positive and supportive framework to do so.

The introduction of clinical governance into the NHS offers the possibility of a shift in culture which could lead to whistle blowing becoming unnecessary. Clinical governance is described as 'a framework which helps all clinicians to continuously improve quality and safeguard standards of care' (RCN 1998, p 2). Crucially, it promises a culture which is 'an improvement-based approach to quality in health care (which) needs to create an enabling culture which celebrates success and learns from mistakes rather than seeking to attribute blame' (RCN 1998, p 3). Another significant change imposed by clinical governance will be that quality of care as well as 'financial probity is the direct responsibility of the Chief Executive, and therefore the Board of NHS Trusts' (Lugon & Secker-Walker 1999, p 1). If the anticipated openness and enablement come to fruition as a consequence of clinical governance, it may well be that nurses' concerns will be dealt with satisfactorily through the normal channels in the health service without the need to whistle blow.

LEGAL RECOURSE FOR WHISTLE BLOWERS

The Public Interest Disclosure Act 1998 has been described as the 'most far-reaching whistleblower law in the world' (Weale 2000). It aims to protect whistle blowers from victimisation and dismissal.

Blowing the whistle on racism in services

119

Ethical and legal framework

Box 5.2.1   Public Interest Disclosure Act 1998

The Act is aimed at protecting whistle blowers from victimisation and dismissal and covers virtually all employees including agency staff, homeworkers, trainees, contractors and professionals in the public, private and voluntary sectors.

It overrides other pieces of legislation and is aimed at providing legal protection for employees who speak out on bad practice in the workplace, be it mismanagement, fraud, victimisation. Revelations may thus be about:

- a criminal act
- a failure to comply with legal obligations
- miscarriage of justice
- danger to health and safety
- any damage to the environment
- an attempt to cover up any of them.

The Act covers the following areas.

- Full protection for almost any worker in the UK against victimisation and dismissal if they whistle blow.
- Bans the use of gagging orders which prevent the whistle blower from speaking out publicly.
- As long as their intention is not malicious, even if the complaining worker's accusations are not proven, they are protected from victimisation.
- Complaining to the police or the media will be permissible if the worker is convinced that revelation to management will lead to a cover-up.
- Whistle blowers who are victimised following a disclosure protected by the Act can take their claim to an employment tribunal for compensation.
- If they are dismissed from work they can apply for an interim order to keep their job, pending a full hearing.

The effectiveness of the legislation in relation to racism and health care is yet to be demonstrated. Roger Kline, national health secretary at the Manufacturing, Science and Finance Union, argues that this will have to be monitored if black and Asian workers are to be protected (Enisuoh 1999). It is impossible to say how Chandra would have fared had she persevered with her complaint and gone public. There are, however, some encouraging reports of whistle blowers receiving compensation for unfair treatment under the new law. Bryan Bladon, a charge nurse who exposed bad practice at a nursing home, received £23 000 after taking his former employer to an industrial tribunal (Weale 2000).

CONCLUSION

This chapter has discussed some of the ethical, professional and legal aspects of whistle blowing in relation to race and health. We have focused our discussion around the case of Chandra, a nurse we assume to be conscientious in her practice but ultimately forced to leave because her concerns were not responded to. Managers have a number of roles to play in relation to whistle blowing. Preventing the conditions which lead to workers feeling concerned is what managers should aspire to. Racist attitudes and behaviours are pernicious to clients/patients and staff and need to be eradicated from health care. The authors are optimistic that an understanding of professional values, clinical governance and the Public Disclosure Act may assist managers in their aspiration towards excellence in care.

References

Baddeley P 1993 The Whistle. Freedom to Care 2:3

Brindle D 1990 Yours sincerely, F G Pink. Guardian, 11 April

Callahan J C (ed) 1988 Ethical issues in professional life. Oxford University Press, Oxford, pp 315–322

Chadwick R, Tadd W 1992 Ethics and nursing practice – a case study approach. Macmillan, Basingstoke

Dobson R 1998 Sick to death of morals. Independent 9 June, p 12

Enisuoh A 1999 Blowing the whistle. Asian Times and Caribbean Times 1 October: 4–5

Guardian 1998 He knew his career would suffer but he had to stop the babies dying. Guardian 30 May, p 5

Health Visitor 1993 Health news – health authority admits unfair dismissal. Health Visitor 66(4):114

Hugill B 1992 Fraud probe after hospital sacks its whistleblower. Observer, 11 October

Hunt G (ed) 1995 Whistleblowing in the health service – accountability, law and professional practice. Edward Arnold, London

Lugon M, Secker-Walker J (eds) 1999 Clinical governance – making it happen. Royal Society of Medicine Press, London

MacPherson W 1999 The Stephen Lawrence inquiry. Stationery Office, London

Royal College of Nursing 1998 Guidance for nurses on clinical governance. RCN, London

Snell J 1992 Whistle-blowing doctor to get back job. Nursing Times 88(46):9

United Kingdom Central Council 1992 Code of professional conduct. UKCC, London

United Kingdom Central Council 1996 Guidelines for professional practice. UKCC, London

Weale S 2000 Is it safe to speak out? Guardian 3 July, pp 8–9

Blowing the whistle on racism in services

Chapter **Six**

Disability: constructing dependency through social policy

Bob Sapey, John Stewart, Jennifer Harris

O V E R V I E W

By chronologically following critiques of the welfare state over 40 years of its most recent history, in this chapter we show how disabled people emerged from being the objects of welfare provision by all-knowing experts to being the objects of welfare production in the post-Fordist world of the informational economy. We examine how the movement of disabled people was able to use the social model of disability to create a real space for themselves and their explanations. The liberation of the social model also provides an insightful critique on the dominant view of disabled people as dependent and as deserving. We argue that what disabled people want is equality of treatment and outcome. The achievement of those basic social rights as part of their civil liberties is still compromised because New Labour's New Deals offer one route only into acceptable non-dependency – paid employment in the formal economy.

INTRODUCTION

People working within the fields of health and social welfare have experienced massive and often continuous change in the way the services are organised and delivered. While it has sometimes been possible to understand the political motivations of government decisions and to make predictions about the outcomes for welfare recipients, this is becoming increasingly difficult as politicians claim to be following a 'third way'. This chapter describes the development of social policy in Britain and examines it in relation to disability services. It goes on to propose ways in which we can make sense of 'third way' politics in order to also make sense of our working situations.

THE SOCIAL ADMINISTRATION TRADITION

Trying to understand how social policies 'on disability' came to be made, what they were intended for or how the implementation of those policies have impacted on the lives of disabled people cannot be achieved without first grasping how our understanding of social policy and administration has changed. Before the First World War the academic discipline of social administration was about the study of the social services. It was created, in the London School of Economics, as handmaiden to training courses for people who intended to work in the statutory and voluntary social services. Hence, in the case of disability, the social administration approach accepted uncritically whatever the benefits and services for disabled people were and merely sought to inform relevant personnel about those provisions and suggest improvements in administration.

Massive may have been the expansion of the social services in personnel and matériel in the postwar euphoria of the Labour government's social reconstruction but the study of social administration remained essentially the same. The focus was concrete and specific. Hence experts would ask, what needs to be changed in this particular policy? (The seminal accounts come from Richard Titmuss, Professor of Social Administration at the London School of Economics from 1951 to 1973, and see, for example, Titmuss 1963 and 1974).

The subject was unashamedly partisan. The point of social administrative study was to advance welfare services by producing information which could be directly used by policy makers and

Disability: constructing dependency through social policy

campaigners who wished to implement changes. But one had to be an evangelist committed to welfare provision which would reduce the 'heavy load of human longing for a better world' (Pinker 1977, p xiv). Furthermore, these doyens of the social administration tradition might have protested that the subject could only be understood in the context of the whole economic, social and political scheme of a particular society but they rarely followed this through in their own researches or analyses. They can be characterised as partial and parochial. Social administration was a very English, and London-based, account of the social services. Seldom did these researchers range further north than Hackney for their evidence. In this tradition social policy was studied in isolation from the theories, perspectives and insights provided by sociology, politics and economics.

Because the leaders of the social administration tradition were Fabians, they shared a belief in the inevitability and rectitude of their cause. Reform was to be gradual and informed by technocratic 'experts' in health or pensions, all to be achieved in the sunshine days of continued economic expansion. Making policies was a rational affair in which the experts revealed needs which would be met by state intervention. In identifying social needs through 'fact-finding' studies, advising government on what policies to implement and being their own advocates for the continued state expansion of welfare, financed through economic growth, the academics of the social administration tradition became enslaved to the state's criteria of what counted as 'success' in the implementation of policies. Critically at this point in the heyday of the late 1960s, although there was a belief in equality, the last people they would ask about whether services 'worked' or were even needed would be the service users themselves.

The key components of the social administration tradition were therefore: a belief that there was a consensus in society around goals in an identifiable field labelled 'social policy'; a rationalist view of how policy is made; and a naive belief in the benign, disinterested character of state institutions. The too-cosy house of social administration collapsed around 1973, principally because the inevitability of economic growth was revealed as a sham by the oil crises. The political nature of social policies had become clear under a Conservative government intent on change. The consensus about welfare aims and objectives vanished as young, vigorous investigators revealed that the welfare state had failed to deliver 'greater equality'. The old experts had predicted that reform of state services would achieve equality of opportunity but it was the welfare state which was providing the new slums in

Ethical and legal framework

high-rise dwellings and on outer estates as old communities were destroyed, literally by demolition. Homelessness was growing at an alarming rate, poverty had not been abolished, the NHS had not brought equality in health care – and so on. Indeed, the very researchers in the social administration tradition, such as Abel-Smith and Townsend, exposed these shortcomings but did not identify their root causes. It was still widely assumed by such traditionalists that more of the same type of welfare medicine would effect a cure.

CRITICAL REAPPRAISALS

Critiques of welfare arose which questioned all the traditional assumptions. The principal critique has been of the structural racism and sexism within the Beveridge Report and the administrative measures which flowed from it (Williams 1989). In part, the Beveridge plan was based on assumptions about the particular contribution which women were meant to make to the economy and the family: 'The attitude of the housewife to gainful employment outside the home is not and should not be the same as that of the single woman. She has other duties' (Beveridge 1942, para 114). The assumption was that married women would be at home looking after male breadwinners and other dependants. It is clear from the Report (pp 108–111) that ' … maternity is the principal object of marriage' and married women were to be treated as dependants of their husbands. Their status as mothers was in the national interest: they had no other.

In a neat turn of phrase which critics have argued wraps patriarchy up with racism Beveridge states: 'In the next thirty years housewives as mothers have vital work to do in ensuring the adequate continuance of the British race and of British ideals in the world' (Beveridge 1942, para 117). However, it is unclear whether, in 1942, Beveridge was referring to Great Britain alone or to the countries which made up the then British Empire. In the midst of the Second World War, before the Allies had won at either Alamein or Stalingrad, it now seems prophetic that Beveridge should have limited his version of patriarchy to 30 years, as the feminist critique began in the 1970s!

The critical edge introduced by feminist and antiracist academics continued to challenge policy changes. In relation to black people, criticism has revolved around the increasing need for service providers to recognise the multiracial contexts within

Disability: constructing dependency through social policy

which the services take place, the limited nature of the efforts to address cultural, linguistic and religious diversity and the dangers of making tokenistic efforts to resolve complex situations (Ahmed 1994, p 119). The short-term funding of specialists to work with black people and the limitation of such a brief only exacerbated inadequate services, rather than tackling the lack of recognition of racism which underpins non-cultural specificity. There are important lessons to be learned from the failure of those initiatives concerning the ideologies underpinning service provision and the ways in which these can never be viewed as value free. Antiracists and feminists have pointed out that these ideologies are biased towards a white ideal and specifically gendered.

The criticisms do not end here as both disabled and older people have claimed that services are provided within a framework which does not recognise structural oppression. Within the context of such criticisms it is likely that the more complicated a person's circumstances and the more oppressive the factors to which a person is exposed, the less likely it may be that service provision could meet needs. The populist notion of successive governments in providing for an imagined majority over the past 50 years has led to these problems of achieving equality of access to services. As social 'problems' became defined into 'needs' for which it was argued there should be a service, in the social administration tradition experts were drafted in to provide a 'specialist' service for whatever particular group had been targeted. This type of crudely reactive strategy has proved unhelpful to say the least, principally because it has been so socially divisive.

Perhaps the clearest example has been in the field of social rented housing. After the war it was intended to be the vehicle for mass housing but the policy did not recognise 'homelessness' as a priority need for rehousing! The majority who were judged to 'need' social rented housing were not homeless. After much traditional social administration-style campaigning, the specialist provision introduced since 1977 prioritised 'homeless families' to such an extent that it could be shown there was hardly any other way of actually being allocated a tenancy in some boroughs. Now 'homelessness' is one priority for housing amongst others. Historically, administrative procedures have allowed 'homeless families' to be stigmatised as queue-jumpers when their housing circumstances were just another version of 'need' – not particularly dissimilar from others in housing need but perhaps more urgent.

Ethical and legal framework

THE FOUNDATIONS OF WELFARE FOR DISABLED PEOPLE

One of the most significant aspects of the self-appraisal with which the social policy/administration academics lashed each other in the late 1970s and 1980s was highly relevant to the emerging disabled people's movement. At last it was being recognised that social services could be neither benevolent nor disinterested over their administration of welfare. In addition, it was also recognised that the 'social problem' focus of traditional social administration had been as ideologically constructed as any other stance. Hence, it followed that all the welfare provisions, from the reforming times of the postwar Labour government down to the 1970s, needed to be critically reappraised. For example, whose perception of the needs of disabled people or even the meaning of disability itself was being served by the extant welfare services for disabled people? The Act, which ostensibly started it off, is in fact very thin on provisions (National Assistance Act 1948, section 29). With regard to welfare, that Act did most of its job in section 1 by abolishing the poor laws! The point here is that having put no serious critical thought into what new 'welfare arrangements for blind, deaf, dumb and crippled persons' might be about, social administrators simply conveyed the medical model of disability (see below) which had served under the poor laws and assumed 'experts' would deal with the intricacies of practice in relation to disabled people. Their thinking was dominated by a focus upon 'impairment'; by the provision of aids and adaptations and by providing institutions – a better class of workhouse. The late 1960s and early 1970s also saw a resurgence of interest in Marxist ideas which undermined the intellectual base of traditional social administration by questioning the possibility of consensus over aims and objectives and the independence of the state in promoting benevolent reforms. Such critical debate was located within the mainstream of sociological study, which itself was emerging from functionalism.

Critics were asking what was the purpose of various welfare measures; whose purposes were being served by them? The service providers of the welfare state began to be characterised as agents of social control, dependency and patriarchy. It is not too far-fetched to suppose that if social administration had not radically reinvented itself it would just have been swept aside by the powerfully explanatory and burgeoning critiques of which feminism is probably the leader, but of which the social model of disability (see below) is certainly another. These new social movements had both

Disability: constructing dependency through social policy

explanatory force and a commitment to welfare very different from the patrician order of traditional social administration.

The 16 desultory sections of Part III of the National Assistance Act 1948, which were supposed to be the foundation of provision for disabled people in the postwar welfare state, had at their heart an ideology that sought to control the extent to which the state should accept responsibility. The nature of the institutional provision, along with the determination of Parliament to ensure that the needs of disabled people were defined by local authorities, represented a clear continuation of the poor law and even subsequent legislation, down to the NHS and Community Care Act 1990, reinforced this position. With his impeccable social administration credentials, Titmuss wrote of this with searing clarity.

> General agreement was reached in Britain during the 1940s that the poor law should be abolished; the philosophy by which it was upheld and the means which it employed were no longer acceptable to the mass of the people. To say this is not, of course, to say that it has been abolished. It can assume another form; acquire another name; reappear in a new dress. As a way of regarding people, the philosophy of the poor law is deeply embedded in the structure of English society. (Titmuss 1954)

While the impetus for segregated forms of care certainly arose from the desire to limit welfare expenditure, it also stemmed from the attitude that disabled people should be the deserving recipients of the benevolence of the day. As Titmuss warned, poor law attitudes could be continuously reconstructed. In 1948, Group Captain Leonard Cheshire formed the Cheshire Foundation with the aim of providing homes and employment for disabled ex-servicemen. Campbell & Oliver (1996) describe the ensuing debate over whether the foundation's efforts should be targeted at building accessible homes or the provision of nursing homes. It settled on the latter with the availability of government funding for that purpose and because it felt that the provision of a total environment in which the *men* could both live and work would be of more help to them. However, within 20 years, any gratitude which may have been present turned to resentment, particularly amongst the newer and younger residents of these institutions. Paul Hunt, who lived in one of the Cheshire Homes and felt his life devalued by his segregation, wrote to *The Guardian* in 1968, trying to make contact with other disabled people who might have similar feelings. The disabled people's movement thus became an organised activity and along with it came an analysis of disability that was to challenge the nature of the welfare state.

MODELS OF DISABILITY

Disability had been viewed traditionally as a medical problem and this was reflected in the definitions agreed by the World Health Organisation.

- *Impairment* – any loss or abnormality of psychological components or anatomical structure or function.
- *Disability* – any restriction or lack (resulting from an impairment) of ability to perform an activity in the manner or within the range considered normal for a human being.
- *Handicap* – a disadvantage for a given individual, resulting from an impairment or disability, that limits or prevents the fulfilment of a role that is normal, depending on age, sex, social and cultural factors, for that individual.

However, this view of disability, based on the concept of disabled people as different and abnormal, was rejected by the Union of Physically Impaired Against Segregation (UPIAS), which had started to articulate the feelings of disabled people that their problems arose primarily from a social reaction to their impairment rather than as a direct result of it. Their alternative definitions explain this as well as rejecting the notions of normality and abnormality.

- *Impairment* – lacking part of or all of a limb, or having a defective limb, organism or mechanism of the body.
- *Disability* – the disadvantage or restriction of activity caused by a contemporary social organisation which takes no or little account of people who have physical impairments and thus excludes them from the mainstream of social activities (UPIAS 1976).

The critique of welfare which arose from the actions of disabled people was developed by a number of disabled academics, notably Finkelstein (1980), Oliver (1983, 1990), Morris (1991) and Barnes (1991). The social model of disability rejected the direct causal relationship between impairment and disability that was central to the individual or medical model and instead redefined disability as a form of social oppression. Barnes (1991) undertook a major study of health, welfare, education, employment, housing, transport, leisure and political life of disabled people in which he concluded that institutional discrimination existed in all parts of British life and that in order to combat this it was essential to introduce antidiscriminatory legislation. He identified the welfare system as

Disability: constructing dependency through social policy

responsible for the economic deprivation of disabled people through its 'excessive bureaucratic regulation and control' (p 228). He went on to say:

> This dependence is compounded by the present system of health and social support services, most of which are dominated by the interests and concerns of professionals who run them and the traditional assumption that disabled people are unable to take charge of their own lives. (p 228)

Even in areas of health provision which might be considered positive, such as rehabilitation, he argued that these were geared to forcing disabled people to adapt to an impossible and hostile environment, placing the responsibility on the individual rather than modifying or removing the barriers to integration. While some effort has been made in recent years to remove the more obvious physical barriers through the provision of, say, ramps for wheelchair access to public buildings, other impediments persist and may have become worse. For example, the health checks on people entering nurse training prevent almost all disabled people from entering this profession, not because they are unable to do the job but because employers perceive impairments as problematic and potentially making them liable for any errors in practice.

IDEOLOGY AND DEPENDENCY

Disabled people are thus subjected to treatment and control by the welfare state that is not applied to all people and would not be tolerated by others. Throughout the various areas of public provision the 'problem' of disability has been 'resolved' by removing disabled people. Segregated education, segregated employment and unemployment, segregated nursing homes and the withholding of certain medical treatments have all formed part of this response to impairment, giving rise to some real doubt as to whose interests the welfare state is actually intended to serve. Finkelstein (1991) took the argument further by questioning the legitimacy of defining the needs of disabled people as welfare. Indeed, it is hard to imagine any government managing to define the access, transport, leisure or employment needs of the rest of the population as welfare issues or that such a position would be accepted by them. So why is it that disabled people are consistently subjected to such regulation of their lives? At the core of this debate is the notion of dependency. We have allowed ourselves to limit, restrict and intervene in the lives of disabled people whilst at the same time making them inhabit a built environment in the image of non-impaired people. We did this in the name of their assumed dependency and then recreated that very dependency by our works.

The debate can be understood in terms of historical tensions between collectivism and anticollectivism (George & Wilding 1985). On this analysis the resulting consensus, characterised as the 'reluctant collectivism' of the Keynesian-Beveridge welfare state, supported an administrative system which provided for those who were unable to participate within the rigours of a capitalist economy, primarily to maintain a level of social cohesion. However, since 1979 through the reborn influence of anticollec-tivist neo-classical liberals (Thatcherites), we were taught to believe that welfare must be strictly controlled. Disabled people were easy to identify as unable to participate within an industrial economy and as a consequence became the recipients or victims of welfare. To some extent they were pitied and considered deserving of welfare help but not of anything which might lead to their inclusion in the mainstream economy. Disabled people became welfare dependants.

GLOBAL FUTURES AND THE THIRD WAY

As we move through the information revolution, the relationships of capital and labour are subjected to new pressures and are in the process of change (Castells 1996). The position of disabled people within this informational economy may also have changed with some gaining greater access to employment through the availability of technology and the changing nature of production. Furthermore, at a political level the impact of this change and the globalisation of capital has led some commentators to begin to talk of a 'third way', suggesting that the simple polarisation of two ideological positions within the nation-state may be an outdated method of analysis. In Britain this has become a reality since the election of New Labour in 1997. Tony Blair has become the first prime minister to openly accept that national politics are limited and subservient to global economic and social forces. The ideologies of the past were important as they determined how the state would be governed but if one accepts that the nation-state can only manage rather than govern, then ideology may be redundant at a national level. The problem for those living through such changes who are engaged in ideologically driven occupations such as welfare is how to predict what this will mean to the services they offer.

131

The lack of certainty and predictability of the future has for some time given rise to theories that might be categorised as postmodernist in that they appear to accept that a greater degree of eclecticism is necessary to explain the world and the way people act or behave within it. Indeed, Darendorf's (1998) recent appeal to Blair to abandon the third way in favour of 101 ways and to end his search for THE big idea might well be a reflection of this thinking. Management too has been urged to forget strategic thinking in favour of managing chaos (Peters 1989) and this has been particularly prominent in British public services where the crisis of change has led to a crisis of confidence amongst those working in them. However, while there may well be 101 ways and a need to manage the chaos that arises from such diversity, it would be wrong to give up on the notions of strategic thinking and planning.

In his analysis of the information revolution and the globalisation of the economy, Castells (1996) argues that no single factor can predict the changes that have occurred or will occur. Rather, change is the product of social, political and technological factors with social and political influences being prominent in determining and shaping technology. Thus what we need to understand is the manner in which technological changes affect the economy and the character of the social and political forces which will shape them in the future. In this sense it is important to understand New Labour's attitude towards governance, as this will affect significantly the regulation of the British economy and hence its social policies.

NEW DEALS

The first three years of the New Labour government have shown that they accept limitations on the scope of their governance, despite implementing a massive overhaul of welfare through the New Deals and Welfare to Work projects. For example, the previous Conservative government's spending plans have been rigorously supported. If the economic policies of the government are to be determined by the needs of global capital then so, of course, will the social ones. Therefore we are unlikely to see any significant increases in welfare spending but are likely to experience considerable redistribution in the existing provisions. Most contentiously, we have already witnessed the transfer of one parent benefit and lone parent premium to childcare provision. This reversal of a previous political stance has been justified on the twin grounds of keeping to the last government's spending plans and encouraging yet more women carers into employment. However, the increase in Child Benefit has been considerable and the Working Family Tax Credit and Childcare Tax Credit are in place. It is known that the body reviewing the Disability Living Allowance has considered replacing cash payments to individual disabled people by local authority services for them (*Independent* 22.12.97). As we have already noted, providing services directly through regulated agencies is a means of ensuring greater control.

In terms of employment the government argues:

> In Labour's first Budget, we raised £3.5 billion to spend on our welfare to work programme. Over the coming months we are extending the New Deal to new groups: the long-term unemployed, partners of the unemployed, and disabled people. There will also be a New Deal for Communities to extend economic opportunity to some of the most deprived areas in the country ... Helping those who cannot work is a mark of a civilised society. The Government believes that those who are disabled should get the support they need to lead a fulfilling life with dignity ... The Labour Government has given to disabled people a right which has been denied to them for too long – the right to work. Many people with a disability or long term illness are simply not in a position to undertake work. Our commitment to their welfare is unwavering. (Labour Party 1998)

These proposals are now under way and currently being reviewed. It has to be said that the initial reaction of disabled people to the intentions behind the proposals has not been ecstatic, with considerable concern voiced by some at the veiled intention to cut disability benefits in the same way that 'redistributive' measures have been applied to single parent benefits.

The Chancellor of the Exchequer's pre-Budget report 2000 points out that only 11% of working-age people on Disability Living Allowance 'are in work or looking for work. The goal of the New Deal for disabled people is to increase the labour force participation rate of this highly disadvantaged group'. Whilst outlining the terms of the Deal, the Chancellor notes that only 5000 people with disabilities, or 30% of those participating, had found work through the Deal by September 2000 (HM Treasury 2000, p 12). The Department of Social Security makes it clear in the policy White Paper *Opportunity for all – one year on* (2000) that the only way disabled people are to be considered is in terms of their employment-ready potential:

Disability: constructing dependency through social policy

> Budget 2000 announced the first stage of work in developing nation wide services to help disabled people find work. We are also taking action to help working people when they first become ill, before they lose touch with their jobs and with the labour market. (DSS 2000, Ch. 3, para. 23)

The only mention of Incapacity Benefit is in terms of 'changes to the benefits system that will help IB claimants return to work'.

The welfare-to-work programme has been supported by setting up the Social Exclusion Unit to consider the plight of people who are believed not to participate in society. Because their notion of 'social exclusion' is primarily work focused, one can ask whether the unit will treat non-participation as the result of external forces or internal motivation. In other words, will the Social Exclusion Unit blame the individual single parent for not finding employment or will they examine the structure of industry, employment and social support in a society that is principally organised around an ideal of the two-parent family? At this point in time the messages from their reports seem to be mixed. On the one hand the economic policies appear to be no different to those of the Conservatives which were clearly aimed at the motivation of the individual, but the actual setting up of the Social Exclusion Unit appears to suggest a broader understanding of the causes of such exclusion. Their actions over the course of this government will therefore provide clear indicators of the direction of welfare.

In terms of disability, it will be of particular relevance to see if the changes the government introduces go any way towards addressing the structural problems in employment that have been identified by disabled people. In this respect New Labour has inherited and appears to be supporting the Disability Discrimination Act 1995. This Act is now the major legislative measure concerning the employment of disabled people, replacing the Disabled Persons (Employment) Act 1944. While it makes discrimination on the grounds of disability in employment illegal, it simultaneously makes it *legal* to discriminate where it would be unreasonable not to (for a comprehensive guide to this issue, see Gooding 1996). Since coming to office New Labour has appointed a group to oversee the 1995 Act. Despite concerns that this might simply amount to the enforcement of a bad piece of legislation, several leading activists of the disabled people's movement now sit on the Disability Rights Commission. Along with observing the actions of the Social Exclusion Unit, it will be important to see how the Disability Rights Commission acts over key issues such as removing the barriers to employment which would make it possible for disabled people to be included within the workforce.

In relation to housing, which is an essential aspect of inclusion for disabled people, the government has announced that it will be amending the building regulations to ensure that in the future, all homes will be built to an accessible standard. This is a significant indicator of New Labour policy because not only does it show its willingness to stand up to deregulatory pressures from the construction industry, it also shows that it is in tune with the demand for structural change to ensure inclusion. 'Accessible' or 'lifetime' homes were first proposed by the United Nations in 1976 but had been ignored by successive governments, yet for disabled people this means a major policy shift from the provision of 'special' housing in selected enclaves to having something more like the same choice as other people.

In a similar move in October 1997, when launching the White Paper *Excellence for all children*, David Blunkett, the Secretary of State for Education and Employment, made clear his opposition to segregated education and announced his intention to reduce the numbers of children in special schools. The initial response of the National Association of School Masters and Union of Women Teachers, however, was to threaten 'not to teach' certain children if integration went 'too far'. It is simply unimaginable that such a threat would ever be made or upheld on the basis of gender, religion, race or virtually any other social division or characteristic of children but in relation to disability, the teachers' stance is accepted by many as 'responsible'. Indeed, while race and sex discrimination laws apply to education, they are specifically excluded from the provisions of the Disability Discrimination Act 1995. The resolve of New Labour to ensure equality of citizenship for disabled people will be judged by the degree to which the Secretary of State ensures that professional pleading does not overrule the educational needs of those disabled children.

POWER RELATIONS

The issue of power is central to the social model analysis of disability. Power is also of crucial significance in the relationships between disabled people, the welfare institutions and the professions which service them. It will be useful, therefore, to draw upon an analysis of power relations to guide our understanding. While Castells' analysis is a macro one, there are aspects of his theoretical perspective that lend themselves to a microanalysis of the relationship between health professions and disabled people.

Disability: constructing dependency through social policy

The theoretical perspective underlying this approach postulates that societies are organized around human processes structured by historically determined relationships of production, experience and power. Production is the action of humankind on matter (nature) to appropriate it and transfer it for its benefit by obtaining a product ... Experience is the action of human subjects on themselves ... It is constructed around the endless search for fulfilment of human needs and desires. Power is that relationship between human subjects which, on the basis of production and experience, imposes the will of some subjects upon others ... Institutions of society are built to enforce power relationships existing in each historical period, including the controls, limits, and social contracts achieved in the power struggles. (Castells 1996, pp 14–15)

As we have argued, disabled people have been excluded from the processes of production and therefore to a great extent from its products. In this sense they have clearly been the victims of power relationships which have sought to exclude them as unproductive. Oliver (1990) argues that economic exclusion and social segregation following the industrial revolution have indeed been the experience of disabled people and that this shapes their perception of their position in society. However, in relation to medicine and health, disabled people have not simply been the victims of power relations but have been treated as the matter of production. Their experience is not just that of powerlessness but of a dehumanising process within the role of a dysfunctional body. This view was given some gruesome administrative credibility by Castle Morpeth District Council in August 1998 when they argued that they were not liable for the funeral expenses of a woman who had died in a private nursing home because:

> Without wishing to appear insensitive, one could argue that from a commercial viewpoint residents of a home are its income-producing raw material. Ergo, from a purely commercial view, deceased residents may then be regarded as being the waste produced by their business. (Thomas 1998)

While the ombudsman described this as far-fetched and insulting, it nevertheless illustrates that such views are held by public officers in organisations and institutions involved in the care of disabled and elderly people (and presumably supported by elected members too). These assumptions are similar to those which have informed so much recent policy – to limit the financial liability of the authority. Similarly, the debate that took place in Bradford social services in August 1998, over whether or not to take into care the unborn child of a disabled woman, was motivated by cost rather than care factors. That welfare measures should have the effect of reducing the lives of disabled people to purely economic factors is hardly surprising bearing in mind that the institutions of capitalism drive the state to implement appropriate modes of social regulation, to maintain or enhance capital's ability to prosper. What we should consider therefore is who actually prospers through the provision of welfare.

While the implementation of certain social policies segregates, or at least excludes, most disabled people and indeed forces some of them to live in institutions, those very institutions have become a mode of production for nursing and medicine. This mode of production is supported by institutional regulations which make it compulsory for disabled people to become the matter of the nursing industry. First, the regulations that govern the registration of nursing homes require a qualified nurse to be in charge of such establishments. Simultaneously, the budgetary and legislative guidance to local authorities, combined with the economics of community care in which institutions are more profitable than home care, ensure that disabled people often have little choice other than to accept a passive role living within such places. While the regulations are framed by people who purport to be concerned with protecting vulnerable people, their control over the definitions of both 'vulnerability' and 'care' results in disabled people being forced to become the matter of nursing for profit. In effect, the regulations that purport to protect people actually imprison them. The professional codes of nursing collude with this process.

Despite a slight trend away from the segregation of younger disabled people (DoH 1996), this industry has expanded and diverted into the production of older disabled people in increasingly more clinical settings. For nursing, therefore, the challenge of working in non-oppressive ways with disabled people must include the recognition of its professional control over such production through its contract with society to maintain disabled people in permanent dependency. Presumably Blair's 'third way' in this instance would need to involve intervention in the social mode of regulation. But just which institutions would achieve this is a further problem as the acceptance of social responsibility without social regulation is radically different from policies which have informed the welfare state this far.

Abortion procedures further typify the regard in which disabled people are held within the medical profession. The Abortion Act 1967 makes it legal to terminate a pregnancy in one of two circumstances: first, if it poses a risk to the mother or her family and second if:

there is a substantial risk that if the child were born it would suffer from such physical or mental abnormalities as to be seriously handicapped. (Section 1(1)(b))

Legislation combined with high-tech screening and the economically partial advice of health personnel produces a eugenicist approach which devalues diversity. This is not an argument against abortion per se but against policies and practices which single out a particular group of people as undeserving of life. In fact, if abortion were available on demand it would remove such structural discrimination although many individuals might still choose on the same grounds.

When the social administration tradition was radically appraised after the late 1970s it became accepted that the subject matter of social policy and its administration should be the whole complexity of social institutions and relationships which meet human need – however they might be financed or ordered. It is not 'the government' who decides how human need should be defined and met, but ourselves. It is important to understand not just the institutional processes but the value base from which they operate and the power they have over the distribution of resources. When applied to welfare services for disabled people, we can readily see that as a group their power was relatively weak, their own command over the distribution of resources slight and hence their status was low. Social policy analysis, critically reconceived, has indeed much to offer the disabled people's movement for it is still concerned with the intimate detail of redistribution but in a sharper, economically aware and politically informed manner.

We have to understand the ideological imperatives which drove Thatcherism and are now driving New Labour at a general level of theorising but such analysis also needs to be grounded in empirical studies providing information about the impact of policies on the lives of real, disabled people. Activists of the disabled people's movement have gradually brought all disabled people and 'disability' itself into the political arena. Abandoning the intellectually cosy world of the medical model with its entailment of hierarchical expert provision and assured 'deserving' status has been hard. Disabled people compete openly now with all the other groups in the scramble for welfare resources. There are no specially reserved places for 'the deserving'. Critical social policy analysis has made that clear to all of us.

Nurses, along with many others – doctors, social workers, occupational therapists, physiotherapists, speech therapists and so

Ethical and legal framework

on – form the workforce of the health and welfare services. They implement and profit from the policies that so often victimise disabled people. The social model of disability provides a powerful and critical analysis of both society and welfare, which can be applied to practice so that welfare professionals can work with, not against disabled people.

CONCLUSION

This chapter has examined how disabled people have been constructed into forms of dependency during the first half-century of the modern welfare state. The chapter opened with a description of the social administration tradition as one which merely described the existing services but then also campaigned for or promoted more of the same. Critical reassessment came with the feminist and antiracist movements of the 1970s, at a time when the economic situation was totally unfavourable to traditional welfareism.

It has been shown how the early notions of 'disability' implicit in the National Assistance Act 1948 were socially constructed from an ideology of dependency on the 'expert' knowledge of service providers with no input from the service user. Focus was entirely on a medicalised notion of 'impairment'.

By the 1970s the new social movement of feminism was overhauling the cosy ideology of a benevolent welfare state. We explained how the disabled people's movement grasped the implications of these critiques. The social model of disability provided a separate, different and powerful explanation of how impairment related to the world – of the built environment and of social relationships in everyday living. Disabled people lacked access in a society created by the non-impaired. And that lack of access was not only to libraries, buses and lavatories, disabled people were discriminated against in the workplace, in school, in higher education and so on.

The differences between the medical model of disability and the social model of disability were explained through their varying interpretations of 'impairment' and its causal relationship with what is meant by 'disabled'. For the disabled people's movement disability is a form of social oppression because, as we show through the work of Barnes, disabled people are made to adapt individually, rather than the barriers to integration being removed by collective action.

Disability: constructing dependency through social policy

139

Next we explained how disabled people are controlled by welfare agencies in ways which would not be tolerated by the non-disabled. The examples taken are from so-called special education.

As our chronology moved into the 1980s we assessed the impact of Thatcherism with its view that all welfare is dependency creating but that some people, if genuine, are more deserving than others. Hence disabled people have a role defined for them as deserving, dependent recipients of expert-defined welfare. We briefly examined how the disabled people's movement resisted this state interpretation, which led us into discussion of their place within the reformulation of welfare under New Labour.

New Labour's 'third way' in British politics accepts the limitations which the globalisation and fragmentation of the markets has visited upon the possibilities for government intervention. We used Castells' explanation of the informational economy to interpret these changes.

The practical, administrative manifestation of these large-scale changes in social and economic relationships has, for us, been Labour's New Deals. There is indeed a New Deal for disabled people and as we show, it boils down to employment in the formal economy. Employment can define a disabled person out of dependency. Those who cannot take up this option and work must be deserving. We have critically examined the actual provisions, insofar as that was possible in the early days of their implementation. Many of the practical measures initiated by New Labour in its early years were around physical access to the built environment, not least of which was the development of the lifetime homes concept – one truly green shoot inspired by the social model of disability. In contradistinction, over the issue of segregated education it would appear the government holds up the exclusionary tendencies of the National Union of Schoolmasters/Union of Women Teachers as a model of responsibility.

We developed arguments from Castells to explain the imbalance of power relationships between the medical professionals and disabled people which we argue leaves disabled people as 'the matter of production' in a postindustrialised welfare system. Examples from nursing care to abortion law and practice show how the lives of disabled people have been reduced to purely economic factors. The radical critique of social policy implied by acceptance and application of the social model of disability is argued to be a liberating force for those care professionals who accept it.

Practice checklist

Readers should consider the following issues which may inform practice.
- The importance of distinguishing clearly what might be meant by 'handicap', 'impairment' and 'disability'.
- Understanding the significance of language as a labelling and stereotyping agent.
- The value of seeing disabled people in the social context of their whole lives, just like everyone else.
- Reflection on the power of governmental policies to influence how people are perceived.
- Consider the role of health and welfare professionals in making and mediating the images we have of disabled people.

Discussion questions

- Explain to a group of sceptical medical colleagues the social model of disability.
- How has the changing understanding of social policy determined the way in which 'disability' and 'disabled people' have been understood since the introduction of the National Health Service?
- Consider how far and in what ways the rights of disabled people are either social rights of citizenship enjoyed by us all or a special case of civil rights.
- As disabled people chase rights, how far do they risk the loss of their status as genuinely deserving of care? Would being employed end the alleged dependency which seems to be the root of disabled people's exclusion?

References

Ahmed S 1994 Anti-racist social work – a black perspective. In: Hanvey C, Philpot T (eds) Practising Social Work. London, Routledge

Barnes C 1991 Disabled people in Britain and discrimination. A case for anti-discrimination legislation. Hurst, London

Beveridge W 1942 Social insurance and allied services. HMSO, London

Campbell J, Oliver M 1996 Disability politics: understanding our past, changing our future. Routledge, London

Castells M 1996 The information age: economy, society and culture: volume 1 – the rise of the network society. Blackwell, Massachusetts

Darendorf R 1998 Ditch the third way, try the 101st. New Statesman 29 May: 21–22

Disability: constructing dependency through social policy

Department of Health 1996 Statistical bulletin: residential accommodation statistics 1996. DoH, London

Department of Social Security 2000 Opportunity for all – one year on. Stationery Office, London

Finkelstein V 1980 Attitudes and disabled people: issues for discussion. World Rehabilitation Fund, New York

Finkelstein V 1991 Disability: an administrative challenge? In: Oliver M (ed) Social work, disabled people and disabling environments. Jessica Kingsley, London

George V, Wilding P 1985 Ideology and social welfare. Routledge and Kegan Paul, London

Gooding C 1996 Blackstone's guide to the Disability Discrimination Act 1995. Blackstone Press, London

HM Treasury 2000 Pre-Budget Report. Stationery Office, London

Labour Party 1998 The Views of the Labour Party. www/labour.org.uk/views/index.html

Morris J 1991 Pride against prejudice. Women's Press, London

Oliver M 1983 Social work with disabled people. Macmillan, Basingstoke

Oliver M 1990 The politics of disablement. Macmillan, Basingstoke

Peters T 1989 Thriving on chaos. Pan, London

Pinker R A 1977 Social theory and social policy. Heinemann, London

Thomas P A 1998 Report of an investigation into complaint No 97/C/4412 against Castle Morpeth Borough Council. Commission for Local Administration in England, York

Titmuss R M 1954 The administrative setting of social service: some historical reflections. Case Conference 1(1): 5–11

Titmuss R M 1963 Essays on the welfare state. Allen and Unwin, London

Titmuss R M 1974 Social policy, Allen and Unwin, London

UPIAS 1976 Fundamental principles of disability. Union of Physically Impaired Against Segregation, London

Williams F 1989 Social policy: a critical introduction. Blackwell, Oxford

Further reading

Corker M, French S (eds) 1999 Disability discourse. Open University Press, Buckingham

Drake R 1999 Understanding disability policies. Macmillan, Basingstoke

Marks D 1999 Disability: controversial debates and psychosocial perspectives. Routledge, London

Morris J 1993 Independent lives: community care and disabled people. Macmillan, Basingstoke

Oliver M, Sapey B 1999 Social work with disabled people. Macmillan, Basingstoke

Priestley M 1999 Disability politics and community care. Jessica Kingsley, London

Thomas C 1999 Female forms: experiencing and understanding disability. Open University Press, Buckingham

Disability & Society (journal), Carfax

Application **6.1**

Bob Sapey, John Stewart, Jennifer Harris

Welfare enactments and disabled people

This chapter lists the most important legislation through which welfare services are provided to disabled people. Where we are quoting from Acts of Parliament, the text is in *italics*. In order to make some of the technical aspects of the Acts easier to understand, we have paraphrased them and here the text is not in italics. We have also used '...' to indicate missing text. In addition, we have added several comments which appear in [square brackets]. Unless stated otherwise, local authority always refers to an English or Welsh social services authority (but not necessarily a Scottish social work authority). We have updated sections of Acts which were amended subsequently.

NATIONAL ASSISTANCE ACT 1948

Part III

Section 21(1)

(a) It shall be the duty of every local authority ... to provide residential accommodation for persons who by reason of age, illness, disability or any other circumstances are in need of care which is not otherwise available to them.

[This is the origin of what is commonly termed 'Part III accommodation'. It should be noted that the duty of the local authority is to provide accommodation only when suitable care is not otherwise available. This does not in itself give local authorities the right to determine the need for residential or nursing home care on the basis of cost.]

Section 21

(2) ... a local authority shall have regard for the welfare of all persons for whom such accommodation is provided.

Six Steps to **Effective Management**

[An important issue here is that the term 'welfare' remains subject to continuous redefinition. Welfare professionals such as nurses and social workers can improve the quality of care by contributing to this redefining.]

Section 29

(1) A local authority shall have power to make arrangements for promoting the welfare of persons to whom this section applies, that is to say persons who are blind, deaf or dumb and other persons who are substantially and permanently handicapped by illness, injury or congenital deformity.

[This section defines disabled people and is later referred to in other enactments as 'section 29' when identifying target recipients. In 1974 the Secretary of State issued a Circular – LAC 13/74 – which extended Section 29(1) by including *'persons suffering from a mental disorder of any description'*. Mental disorder is defined by section 1(2) of the Mental Health Act 1983 as *mental illness, severe mental impairment, mental impairment and psychopathic disorder.*]

(4) The range of services that local authorities can provide under this Act are:
a. Informing people of services available.
b. Teaching people to overcome the effects of disability.
c. Providing workshops and hostels.
d. Providing home-work.
e. Helping people to sell their home-work.
f. Providing recreation.
g. Keeping registers.

[In practice, apart from registers, most of this has been superseded by subsequent legislation, in particular the Chronically Sick and Disabled Persons Act 1970.]

Part IV

Section 47

(1) The following provisions of this section shall have effect for the purposes of securing the necessary care and attention for persons who –
(a) are suffering from grave chronic disease or, being aged, infirm or physically incapacitated, are living in insanitary conditions, and
(b) are unable to devote to themselves, and are not receiving from other persons, proper care and attention.
(2) If the medical officer of health certifies in writing to the appropriate authority that he is satisfied after thorough inquiry and consideration that the interests of any such person as aforesaid residing in the area of the authority or for preventing injury to the health of, or serious nuisance to, other persons, it is necessary to remove any such person as aforesaid from the premises in which he is residing, the appropriate authority may apply to the court of summary

jurisdiction having jurisdiction in the place where the premises are situated for an order under the next following subsection.

[The next subsection then permits the court to order the officer of the appropriate authority to remove the person ... to a suitable hospital or other place ... and to detain and maintain him/her there. An Amendment Act of 1951 made removal even easier, on the certification of the medical officer of health and another medical practitioner alone if *'in their opionion it is necessary in the interests of that person to remove him without delay'*. This power of detention is without the same rights of appeal that exist in the Mental Health Act 1983 or in criminal legislation.]

CHRONICALLY SICK AND DISABLED PERSONS ACT 1970

Section 1

(1) It shall be the duty of every local authority ... to inform themselves of the number of persons to whom ... section 29 ... applies within their area and of the need for the making by the authority of arrangements under that section for such persons.

[It should be noted that this does not require the keeping of registers, yet many local authorities continue to do so which means that they are unlikely to know the needs of people who have not made contact with them.]

(2) Every such local authority –
(a) shall cause to be published ... general information as to the services provided under ... section 29 ... which are for the time being available in their area; and
(b) shall ensure that any such person ... who uses those services is informed of any other of those services provided by the authority (whether under such arrangements or not) which in the opinion of the authority is relevant to his needs and of any services provided by any other authority or organisation which in the opinion of the authority is so relevant and of which particulars are in the authority's possession.

[This means that local authorities must act as a source of information on services for disabled people. However, while they are not obliged to find out what is available, they must pass on any information that they have been told about. This allows other agencies in both the statutory and independent sectors to have their services advertised to disabled people.]

Section 2(1)

Where a local authority ... are satisfied in the case of any person to whom ... section 29 ... applies who is ordinarily resident in their area that it is necessary in order to meet the needs of that person for that authority to make arrangements for all or any of the following matters, namely –

(a) practical assistance in the home;
(b) wireless, television, library or similar recreational facilities;
(c) lectures, games, outings or other recreational facilities;
(d) travelling to participate in any services provided under section 29;
(e) works of adaptation to the home or any additional facilities designed to secure her/his *greater safety, comfort or convenience*;
(f) holidays;
(g) meals;
(h) telephone and special equipment necessary to use a telephone,

then, ... it shall be the duty of that authority to make those arrangements.

[This section provides the basis for most community care services, in particular personal care and aids/adaptations. While local authorities are under a duty to provide these services, this is limited by budgetary constraints. It should also be noted that it is for the local authority to decide if the various services are needed. This allows the local authority and its officers to act in more or less empowering ways, depending on motivation.]

DISABLED PERSONS (SERVICES, CONSULTATION AND REPRESENTATION) ACT 1986

Section 4

When requested to do so by –
(a) a disabled person, or...
(b) any person who provides care for him in the circumstances mentioned in section 8,
a local authority shall decide whether the needs of the disabled person call for the provision by the authority of any services in accordance with section 2(1) of the 1970 Act (provision of welfare services).

[Some local authorities had tried to avoid their duty under the 1970 Act by delaying the assessment of need. They argued that if they did not know the needs of an individual they were free of any responsibility or duty to meet them. This section was intended to rectify that loophole. Sections 5 and 6 also required social services authorities and education authorities to ensure that any child with special needs is assessed when they leave school, to see if they are entitled to services under the 1970 Act.]

Section 8

(1) Where –
(a) a disabled person is living at home and receiving a substantial amount of care on a regular basis from another person (who is not a

*person employed to provide such care by any body in the exercise of
its functions under any enactment), and*
*(b) it falls to a local authority to decide whether the disabled person's
needs call for the provision by them of any services for him under any
of the welfare enactments,*
*the local authority shall, in deciding that question, have regard to the
ability of that other person to continue to provide such care on a
regular basis.*

[This was the first time carers were mentioned in any legislation in
the UK. They are defined by section 8(1)(a) as anyone not employed
by statutory agencies, directly or indirectly, to provide care. The
intention of section 8(1)(b) was to prevent local authorities refusing
services simply because people had carers but to consider the ability
of the carer to continue to care. Again, this is a significant issue over
which welfare professionals have a lot of influence through their
assessments of care relationships.]

Section 10

*Where any enactment provides for the appointment or co-option to
any council, committee or body of one or more persons with special
knowledge of the needs of disabled persons, such appointment or
co-option shall only be made after consultation with such organisation
or organisations of disabled people as may be appropriate in each
case.*

[This refers to people appointed to local authority committees. The
importance of this section is that it requires local authorities to
consult with organisations **of** rather than **for** disabled people. These
organisations are defined by the British Council of Disabled People as
those that are constitutionally controlled by disabled people, e.g. this
would include the Spinal Injuries Association but exclude SCOPE.]

CHILDREN ACT 1989

Schedule 2, Part 1

6. Every local authority shall provide services designed –
*(a) to minimise the effect on disabled children within their area of
their disabilities; and*
*(b) to give such children the opportunity to lead lives which are as
normal as possible.*

[This Act took over the provision of services to disabled children. On
a positive note the above description is much broader than the list of
services in the 1970 Act, but at the same time many local authorities
began to prioritise child protection services over services to disabled
children.]

NATIONAL HEALTH SERVICE AND COMMUNITY CARE ACT 1990

Section 46

(3) In this section – ...
'community care services' means services which a local authority may
provide or arrange to be provided under any of the following
provisions –
(a) Part III of the National Assistance Act 1948;
(b) section 45 of the Health Services and Public Health Act 1968;
(c) section 21 of and Schedule 8 to the National Health Service Act
1977; and
(d) section 117 of the Mental Health Act 1983;

[The importance here, apart from the obvious definitions, is to note that the 1990 Act did not create any new services.]

Section 47

(1) ... where it appears to a local authority that any person for whom
they may provide or arrange for the provision of community care
services may be in need of any such services, the authority –
(a) shall carry out an assessment of his needs for those services;
and
(b) having regard to the results of that assessment, shall then
decide whether his needs call for the provision by them of any such
services.

[This reemphasises the duty of the local authority to assess the needs of, amongst others, disabled people.]

(2) If at any time during the assessment of needs ... it appears to a
local authority that he is a disabled person, the authority –
(a) shall proceed to make such a decision as to the services he requires
as is mentioned in section 4 of the Disabled Persons (Services,
Consultation and Representation) Act 1986 without his requesting
them to do so under that section; and
(b) shall inform him that they will be doing so and of his rights under
that Act.

[The intention of this is to make it obligatory for local authorities to offer an assessment of need to services provided under the 1970 Act whenever they think a person might have an entitlement to any of those services.]

(3) This places a duty on local authorities to inform health and
housing authorities if they think any of their clients might need their
services.

COMMUNITY CARE (DIRECT PAYMENTS) ACT 1996

Section 1

(1) Where –
(a) an authority have decided ... that the needs of a person call for the provision of any community care services, and
(b) the person is ... specified ... by the Secretary of State, the authority may, if the person consents, pay him the whole, or such part as they think fit, of the cost of his securing the provision of any of the services for which they have decided his needs call.

[This gives local authorities the power to make direct payments to disabled people, in order to permit them to purchase their own community care services instead of, or in conjunction with, services provided or purchased by the authority. The disabled person has to request this and local authorities do not have to agree, but it is widely agreed within the disabled persons' movement that this is a positive way of changing the power relations within the care relationship. At the moment this provision does not apply to older people.]

Welfare enactments and disabled people

Chapter **Seven**

Ageism and the law

Lesley Wade

OVERVIEW

The concept of ageism and the statutory power to avoid it appears ambivalent. Therefore the chapter begins by highlighting some prejudices towards older people and uses the Registered Home Act 1984 as a vehicle to exemplify the misinterpretation and irregularities this well-intentioned act created on behalf of older people. The chapter reiterates the need for skilled nursing assessment and highlights some of the key inequalities towards minority elderly groups. Particular attention is paid to the law as it relates to older people's mental health. The chapter concludes by addressing the concept of the 'corruption of care' which can be avoided by confronting ageism as a manager. Our knowledge of the law, the style of management we adopt and the way we actively become involved at all levels, from hands-on care to policy making, can contribute to the avoidance of ageism.

> ### Objectives
>
> This chapter explores the following themes and issues:
> - societal and institutional prejudices towards older people
> - anomalies and inconsistencies within the law towards older people living in care homes
> - specific inequalities towards minority ethnic elders
> - recognising a culture where there is a 'corruption of care'
> - confronting ageism.

Ethical and legal framework

INTRODUCTION

The professional and general media carry endless reports of failing in health and social care towards older people. Remedies are sought in punishing the nurse or carer, removing the manager or introducing new codes to supplement the enforcement of law. This chapter argues that discrimination towards older people pervades our society and laws and is made manifest by the increasing complexities of community care and the divisions between health and social care. Caught between piecemeal legislation, the older person can be forgotten.

PREJUDICES ABOUT POPULATION GROWTH

People are living longer and the number of older people in the UK is increasing. The government actuary's National Population Project (OPCS 1998) shows that the total population of the UK is expected to rise by 2020 and then decrease slightly by 2050. During the same period, expectation of life at birth is projected to increase from 73.9 years for males and 79.2 years for females in 1994 to 77.7 years and 82.6 respectively by 2020. The size of the very old frail section of the population is projected to rise the most rapidly, with the proportion over 75 years estimated to increase from the current 4 million to 5 million by 2020.

Therefore the ageing of the population has important implications for the health care manager, not least in financing and providing long-term care. If morbidity levels remain the same or rise, the number of people who are chronically sick or disabled can be expected to grow. It must be emphasised, however, that the supposed 'demographic time bomb' concept is not justifiable.

Most older people are presently able bodied and of sound mind, although with advancing years there may be increased dependency. From the viewpoint of law, it is this potential dependency allied with problems in decision making that make this group vulnerable. This vulnerability coupled with stereotyping and prejudices towards older people in society is known as ageism (Butler 1963). Ageism can take many forms; it can be either intentional, as in rationing of health care, or, more commonly, unintentional, due to a lack of knowledge and a complete lack of understanding of older adults' needs.

Prejudice towards older people can therefore be seen to operate not only on an individual basis (health care managers may

Ageism and the law

recognise this when they deal with aspects of abuse and misconduct) but also at policy-making levels. Therefore those that interpret the law are just as likely to be exposed to the effects of ageism
and there has been a call for a revaluation of attitudes towards
older people, based on the report *Fit for the future* (Kohln 1998).
Within this paper reference is made to values and attitudes
towards older people shaped by an appreciation that:

- the older population should not be viewed negatively but as a
  major achievement of the 20th century
- old age should be seen as a distinct phase of life which brings
  new opportunities and developments for both individuals and
  society. Older people have considerable assets of time and
  experience contributing to intergenerational interactions,
  within families and wider communities
- social inclusion should be a goal for ensuring opportunities for
  all citizens to participate fully in society, regardless of age,
  gender, ethnicity or socioeconomic group
- policies and practices should reflect the principle of age neutrality and should not use age as a basis for discrimination
- strategies must focus on maintaining and enhancing what older
  people are able to do, rather than what they cannot do
- promoting positive values and attitudes should be part of
  public policy and law.

If, like myself, you are a manager within a health care setting these
values and attitudes, which may seem obvious to you, may not
seem so obvious to fellow colleagues or others in society.

Interestingly, older people within the UK do not have a separate
body of law reserved for them alone. Older people as citizens have
exactly the same rights and access to care as anybody else. Many
feel that a separate body of law dealing solely with older people
would be itself discriminatory and self-destructive. However, the
sea change that has led to an emphasis on community care, especially with a focus on long-term care of the elderly, demonstrates
inadequacies. And whilst it would be discriminatory to have a
separate body of law dealing with older people, many fields of law
need to be modified and enhanced to cater for the diverse needs of
this large group.

THE ROLE OF THE LAW

The role of the law in assisting older people can be divided into
three areas.

Ethical and legal framework

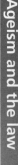

- To protect the individual from exploitation, neglect or abuse, whether physical, mental or financial.
- To enhance the quality of the individual's life by either providing support or enabling decision making.
- To enforce duties owed by society to the individual (Ashton 1995).

This is a very wide remit and health care managers, whether in the increasing independent sector or public sectors, need to use their knowledge of old age to ask a number of questions.

- How can the law protect the vulnerability of such a large heterogeneous group of people?
- Who interprets the law and what is the influence of changing governmental policies and boundary disputes between different professional groups?
- How far can the law support and improve the quality of older people's lives through 'enforcing powers'?

As a manager within an independent care home, the complexities and anomalies within the law affect my everyday practice. As a lecturer in gerontology and practitioner, the impact of provision of care by whom, to whom, has been greatly influenced by the Registered Home Act 1984. Providing care and working within that act makes one aware of some of the well-intentioned aspects of law which need urgent modification.

LONG-TERM CONFUSION AND THE LAW: THE REGISTERED HOME ACT 1984

More than 500 000 older people in the UK live in some form of institutional setting (Hall 1996), the majority in private nursing or residential care homes. The desirability of older people residing within these homes and the quality of this accommodation has become an emotive subject. Individual horror stories involving neglect or abuse of vulnerable older people appear frequently in the press yet legislation on care homes has been in place for some time, laying down minimum quality standards and actual requirements supported by law which should at least guarantee decent living conditions.

If we examine the Registered Home Act 1984 and its effects, what emerges is a well-meaning but outdated piece of legislation that does not take into account contemporary changes related to the provision and quality of care. The Act consolidated various pieces of care legislation dating back to the 1948 National Assistance Act.

Six Steps to **Effective Management**

The Residential Care Home Regulations 1984, together with the Nursing Home Regulations and Mental Nursing Home Regulations of 1984, are the key legislative vehicles ensuring that quality and minimum standards are in place and maintained. However, within these regulations there is scope for variation and interpretation of standards. Interpretation is presently left to the local registration units for nursing homes and residential homes. From a nurse manager's perspective, several thorny issues emanate from turf wars between health and social services, robust and confrontational inspection processes and the dilemma of working within ever-decreasing budgets.

The confusion in long-term care is exemplified by the Pamela McCoughlan case (*Times*, 20 July 1999).

Case study 7.1   The Pamela McCoughlan case

Paralysed from the waist down after a car accident in 1971, Pamela was promised a home for life at a NHS rehabilitation centre. However, a decision was taken by North and East Devon Health Authority to close the home and to find her alternative accommodation in the care of the social services.

The case illustrated the problem of whether nursing was health care or social care. In July 1999 the case went to the High Court. The detailed examination concluded that:

● the Secretary of State could exclude some nursing services from the service provided by the NHS. Such services could then be provided as a social or care service rather than a health service. In simple terms, McCoughlan's nursing care could be given within the social service package of care within her new accommodation
● the major catch was that this nursing service, if part of the social service package of care, would have to be paid for by the person concerned, unless their resources deemed them exempt.

The crux of the matter was that this form of nursing service, as part of the social services, was subject to the same regime of payment as other social services. The ethical considerations of a promise of a home for life and the Human Rights Act 1998 swayed the case. The court ruled that North and East Devon Health Authority was wrong to close Mardon House where the resident had a home for life. However, it also stated that the NHS was entitled to shift responsibility for long-term nursing care onto local authorities. As the *Nursing Times* has indicated, the decision seems to have thrown up more questions than it answered. As Merryn Kohler, head of public affairs at Help the Aged, has stated, 'We are not sure where the boundaries lie' (Kohler 1999).

Significantly, the Residential Care Homes Regulations 1984 emphasised that the first consideration must be to safeguard the individuality of residents and that any decision making on behalf of the individual had to be shaped by their diverse needs.

It is important that we as health care managers, whether in residential, nursing, domiciliary or dual registered homes, critically analyse the Act and its effectiveness. All managers will be confronted by the parts of the Act often quoted to support requirements that have to be complied with. These are public documents available at central libraries, inspection units and on the World Wide Web. Regulation 10 of the Act is an example which is often quoted within inspection reports. It discusses the facilities and services to be provided and includes phrases such as:

- by day and night suitably qualified and competent staff in numbers adequate for the well-being of the residents
- reasonable day and nighttime accommodation and space
- adequate and suitable furniture, bedding, curtains, floor coverings and other equipment
- sufficient washing facilities
- adaptations and facilities for physically handicapped residents
- suitable, varied, nutritious food
- suitable arrangements for the recording, safekeeping, handling and disposal of drugs
- suitable arrangements for recreation and if need be training of residents
- arrangement for residents to receive medical and dental services.

All the above must be interpreted relative to the size, number, gender and condition of the residents.

It can be seen that the Act focuses on physical standards, although the social services inspectorate has addressed the importance of basic values that underpin individuality and the diverse needs of older people. To supplement the Act and recognise the unique individuality of the person, guidelines and codes of practice are used. The most important guidelines, *Homes are for living in* (DHSS 1989), stress issues such as:

- *dignity* – recognising the intrinsic value of people
- *independence* – the opportunity to act and think without reference to others and having the opportunity to take a degree of calculated risk
- *rights* – all older people within any care home continue to have all the rights and responsibilities of citizenship, having a voice in how that institution is run.

Ageism and the law

These underpinning values are themselves not enshrined in law. For nurses, guidelines for professional practice were drawn up by the UKCC under the powers of the Nurses, Midwifes and Health Visitors Acts 1979 and 1996. The code sets out:

- the value of registered practitioners
- your responsibilities to represent and protect the interests of patients and clients
- what is expected of you. (UKCC 1996)

In a recent review of the legislation related to long-term care of older people (Better Regulation Task Force 1998), a number of recommendations were suggested, emanating from the Burger Report (1997) and assisted by salient points made by the RCN (1996) (particularly about incorrect assessment of older people's needs and placements). This is a reaction to the growing realisation that the Registered Care Home Acts and Community Care Act of the 1980s contain anomalies and inconsistencies. One of the major criticisms of the Homes Act is that it creates two parallel systems, one for nursing and one for residential care, that almost duplicate one another. However, the demarcation between the two is not at all clear; the responsibility for personal care and professional care crosses professional boundaries and, as we have seen with the McCoughlan case, budgets. One of the great anomalies is that the concept of nursing is not defined at all!

The dilemma of what is personal care (the extension of care that would be provided by a relative) and what is the undefined nursing care has considerable ethical, financial and professional consequences.

THE NEED FOR CORRECT NURSING ASSESSMENT

The RCN has emphasised the need for correct assessment of older people. Dialogue between nursing home and residential care home owners questions some of the social workers' assessments of older people. They are only too aware, however, that many assessments are budget driven, such as that which classified a 62-year-old woman weighing 4 stone 4 lbs with chronic obstructive airway disease, needing oxygen therapy, as not in need of nursing care. The RCN emphasises that an assessment should include:

- obtaining a comprehensive biography about the person
- assessing the older person's overall health status
- assessing and integrating the physical, mental and psychomotor functioning (Ford et al 1999).

Clearly the scope of the Registered Homes Act 1984 is insufficient and there is a need to review professional practice in the light of older people in institutions, especially within the community.

Clearly, inconsistencies and idiosyncratic behaviours will occur when nursing homes and residential care homes are subject to widely differing licensing regimes whilst other areas, such as domiciliary care supported by the statutory sector, presently go unregulated. Inconsistencies and varied interpretations are a major concern for managers within the independent sector. Differing interpretations in different regions, authorities or even within local government departments themselves regarding fire, space, staffing levels and staffing competencies all create misunderstanding and distrust and waste time and money.

For a manager, the key points that cause tension emanating from the Act of 1984 are:

- a lack of clarity about what constitutes a mandatory requirement as opposed to a recommendation; in other words, what is statutory and what is voluntary
- the ability of local authorities and other care purchasers to set requirements in excess of those applied by those who provide the care
- the ambiguity of terms such as 'fit person', 'standards' and 'codes of practice'.

The Department of Health has set out a number of standards to improve the care of older people in homes, as outlined in the *National Service Framework for older people,* published on 27 March 2001 (DoH 2001).

Setting up a new complaints procedure for nursing homes, John Hutton, Health Minister, stated:

> The government is committed to making horror stories of badly run homes a thing of the past. Today's consultation sets out the national baseline for performance and regulation as well as setting its rules for acceptable standards with enforceable, national standards and national rules. (Hutton 1999)

The minister also highlighted the need for properly trained staff and high-calibre management.

157

INEQUALITIES AND INCLUSIONS

Better Government for Older People is a new national strategy involving numerous agencies, aiming to provide people with clearer, more accessible information on their rights, more say in and simplified access to services and improved linkage between agencies. This is a response to a number of reports on the impact community care has had on older people. The findings suggest that care was targeted at more heavily dependent older people with some notable inequalities of access to care. Problems particularly revolved around ethnic minority groups and older adults with mental health needs.

Ethnic minority groups

Ageist attitudes towards older people from the Commonwealth, including Asia and now some East European states, have been recognised for some 15–20 years (Blakemore & Boneham 1994). The false assumption that ethnic minority groups care for older people collectively has been torn asunder by work carried out by Blakemore & Boneham (1994) with older Caribbean and Asian communities located throughout the British Isles. Recent work by Tarek Quershi (1998) examining a study of Bangladeshi elders in London identified that problems existed for this section of the elderly population in the areas of:

- education
- religion
- family structures
- employment
- concepts like voluntary work
- housing
- health participation
- concepts of citizenship
- intergenerational relations
- racism
- elder abuse
- social isolation.

Quershi's report echoes the findings of a report by the Standing Conference on Ethnic Minority Senior Citizens (1994). This study not only highlighted the issues raised 3 years on but linked with the Commission for Racial Equality to request a formal response from the government, which has not been forthcoming.

158

At local level many health and social services have responded to the issues of inequalities, exclusion and access to health care for ethnic groups. The concept that ethnic groups care for their own elders has been gradually whittled away but we cannot as managers ignore the double jeopardy of being from an ethnic minority and being older within our society and that services need to be developed in a more culturally sensitive manner.

Autonomy and the law

How far our current laws observe or preserve older people's autonomy in regard to a number of important aspects of life – treatment decisions, informed consent, money and property matters – depends upon whether the individual can make or has made an anticipatory choice which has been clearly established. If this is so, the medical practitioner is then bound to follow this, even after clients become incapable of expressing their wishes.

If there is any doubt about aspects of care and choice, doctors are protected by the doctrine of implied consent and may give treatment designed to preserve life, assist recovery or ease suffering.

Mental health

The concept of mental impairment refers to a state of arrest or incomplete development of the mind which includes significant impairment of intelligence and functioning and is associated with abnormal aggressive or seriously irresponsible conduct on the part of the person concerned.

Any individual of whatever age may develop a mental illness that brings them within the scope of the mental health legislation.

Legal principles are challenged by a person's descent into dementia. The law aims to preserve the autonomy of dementia patients, protecting them against injuries to themselves and others and limiting victimisation by others.

The Mental Health Act 1983 in its amended form is the current health legislation and applies to persons suffering from a mental disorder as a 'patient'. The Act provides for the compulsory admission to and detention in hospital, medical treatment in hospital without consent and the review of such detentions. Although with regard to older people these powers are only exercised in a minority of cases, it is important to take note of issues of guardianship and the power of attorney.

Ageism and the law

Guardianship

Under the Mental Health Act in its present form, guardianship is a lesser and more appropriate form of intervention than detention in hospital for older people with mild but significant mental disorders. It is distinct from guardianship of minors and is known as 'statutory guardianship'. The powers of guardians are subject to significant limitations and this has dissuaded authorities and individuals from using guardianship more frequently.

The guardian has three main powers:

● to ensure that the patient resides at a specific place
● to ensure that the patient attends at a place and time specific for the purpose of treatment
● to provide access to the patient at the patient's residence to any medical practitioner or other approved person.

All these are difficult to achieve whilst trying to maintain the rights and autonomy of the older person. Family dynamics and interactions play a central role within the interpretation and enactment of the legislation.

Power of attorney

A power of attorney is a document whereby a person (the donor) gives another person (the attorney) power to act on their behalf. It must be executed as a deed by or in the presence of the donor. Legislation in 1985 created enduring powers of attorney (EPAs) which remain valid notwithstanding the donor's subsequent incapacity to manage their own affairs. EPAs provide a practical, inexpensive way in which older or infirm people may anticipate incapacity. An EPA may be general or specific in its terms. The donor may place restrictions or conditions on the power, for example dealing with property.

THE AVOIDANCE OF AN ABUSIVE CULTURE

The chapter began by assuming that managers, who are still drawn from the rank and file of professional practice, have a positive attitude towards older people. However, reports on abuse echo the work of Kayser-Jones (1992) who found there were still issues of infantilisation, depersonalisation and dehumanisation within all aspects of elderly care. Managers' attitudes can often also be

Ethical and legal framework

disclosed as they concur with age-related rationing of health and social care.

This unwitting type of ageism and unawareness in the development of abusive practices is the most commonplace form of discrimination the manager is likely to encounter.

There is currently no one single definition of elder abuse. Because no single protective piece of applicable legislation exists, the Law Commission has published proposals for legal reform drawing on the child protection model. However, questions are raised regarding the suitability of the approach, given the intrinsic social and legal differences between children and adults.

With regard to preventive measures, Eastman (1998) suggests that there are four key blockages that may help to account for managerial ineffectiveness leading to the continued violation of vulnerable people:

- negative stereotypes of and attitudes towards older people
- ignorance of what constitutes abuse
- denying that abuse has occurred
- fear, especially avoiding confrontation.

Various factors can be seen to contribute towards an abusive culture, especially within institutions.

- An inappropriate power balance at all levels of care, inclusive of the client.
- Staff friction based on conflicting positions about progressive and traditional regimes.
- High staff turnover.
- Low staff turnover.
- Shoddy surroundings and work environment.
- Fear of complaints, audits or inspection reports.
- A number of minor incidents that establish a pattern.
- Uncertainty in the team you are leading regarding your aims and objectives.

Eastman uses the phrase 'corruption of care' whereby managers turn a blind eye to what goes on providing the 'work' continues to function in an outwardly acceptable fashion (Wardhaugh & Wilding 1993). Managers often become so disengaged from reality that they lose sight of the older person as a human being, failing to reorganise their individual responsibility to maintain the dignity and uphold the rights of the elderly. Symptoms of this inappropriate management are demonstrated through statements such as:

Ageism and the law

161

Six Steps to **Effective Management**

- It's not really my responsibility
- I have to keep complaints 'in house' and contained
- I'm too busy
- It's not as bad as that
- Let's look at damage limitation here
- It will reflect badly on me and harm the department's reputation.

One of the key issues to raise is the refusal of managers to recognise inequalities and diversity and confront ageism.

Over the last 15 years there has been a fundamental change within the psychology of health work and particularly in its organisational culture. Eastman sees that organisational rewards that focus on macho management, tough decision making and keeping costs down have reduced the existence of previous caring values. This, combined with the fear of redundancy and being seen as ineffective, has fostered a non-confrontational style. A blame culture has emerged and living and working within such an environment, which already has a high degree of emotional labour, deters whistle blowing. The consequence of this is that often confrontation is ineffective or is transferred inappropriately.

CONFRONTING AGEISM AS A MANAGER

Due to ageism, the older person is vulnerable to all the myriad forms of abuse and dependent on managers to create a culture that is free of abuse. The qualities of effective managers include the following.

- Self-confidence and positive self-image.
- Perception of staff and older people as having worth.
- Well-organised and planned work priorities.
- They confront bad practice.
- They are aware of who blocks them.
- They are supportive and praise disclosure.
- They do apologise.
- They seek advice.
- They vary their decision making.
- They are effective at confrontation.

Despite major improvements within health and social care, forms of discriminatory practice continue to exist. The style of management we adopt and our knowledge of the law contribute to the avoidance of ageism. The RCN's recommendations to managers of nursing homes endorse the need for a culture of quality which focuses on educational updates, appropriate staffing levels and developing staff with strong leadership qualities who in turn favourably influence standards of care (RCN 1996).

CONCLUSION

We will all experience the consequences of being old and at the bottom of the social pecking order. Those who escape some of the negative aspects of ageing – relatively few – are the better off and better educated. Old people are frequently referred to as burdens on society. Such attitudes pervade our actions, language and even our political decisions. Our capacity to distance ourselves from what appears to be 'different', especially related to old age, allows us to disconnect. This deeply rooted undervaluing of the aged and ageing and its knock-on effects, especially abuse, encourage the notion that older people are a problem. Managers at all levels within the health service need to ask what part they can play in challenging negative perceptions about ageing. We are all likely to become old, so there is at least an investment for us in making life better.

Practice checklist

Readers should consider the following issues which may inform practice.

- There is a need to reassess the division between health and social care and the effect it has had on older people.
- We need to consider how far the law can support and improve the quality of care through enforcing powers.
- Consider the outcomes if you are an older person who contradicts known stereotypes.
- We need to reexamine the culture that may produce a corruption of care, examine recent UKCC misconduct hearings or select care homes that have been examined within local authority tribunals.

Ageism and the law

Discussion questions

- The combination of undertraining, inappropriate environments and increasing dependency of older people can lead to discrimination and even abusive practices towards older people.
- Within your area of practice, develop a training programme that assists in avoiding abuse. How would you evaluate this?
- The concept of empowerment within the older community crosses many age groups, personal freedoms and social responsibilities. Consider the issues surrounding empowerment for a selected ethnic minority, a residential care home committee or a dementing older person.
- Although Mrs Althorp is mentally alert you notice that her daughter handles her pension book, which is signed by her mother each week and given over. When next you visit Mrs Althrop in hospital after a fall, she is short of essential items. She has no soap or squash, no jewellery or personal belongings. How would you discuss this issue with her daughter? How far can the nurse/manager get involved within family dynamics?

References

Ashton G 1995 Elderly people and the law. Butterworth, London

Better Regulation Task Force 1998 Long term care. Central Office of Information, London

Blakemore K, Boneham H 1994 Age, race and ethnicity – a comparative approach. Open University Press, Buckingham

Burger T 1997 The regulation and inspection of social services. Department of Health/Welsh Office, London

Butler R N 1963 The life review: an interpretation of reminiscence in the aged. Psychiatry 26:66–76

Department of Health 2001 National Service Framework for older people. Stationery Office, London

DHSS 1989 Homes are for living in. Department of Health and Social Services Inspectorate, London

Eastman M 1998 Why and when institutions do not work. In: Jack R (ed) Residential versus community care. Macmillan, Basingstoke

Ford P, McCormack B, Nazarko L 1999 Ageing matters. RCN, London

Hall J 1996. Cited in Redfern S, Ross S 1999 Nursing older people, 3rd edn. Churchill Livingstone, Edinburgh

Hutton J 1999 Regulating national standards. Seminar, 11th October, London

Ethical and legal framework

Kayser-Jones R 1992 Understanding elderly abuse: a training manual for helping professionals. Longmans, London

Kohler M 1999 Nursing homes. Nursing Times 1(3):5

Kohln E 1998 Fit for the future: the prevention of dependency in later life. Continuing Care Conference, London, E Lilly & Co.

Office of Population Censuses and Surveys 1996 National population project. HMSO, London

Quershi T 1998 Living and growing old in Britain. Centre for Policy on Ageing, London

RCN 1996 Nursing homes: nursing values. Royal College of Nursing, London

Standing Conference on Ethnic Minority Senior Citizens 1994 Geriatric Medicine 28:11–13

United Kingdom Central Council 1996 Guidelines for professional practice. UKCC, London

Wardhaugh J, Wilding P 1993 Towards an exploration of the corruption of care. Criticial Social Policy 13(37):117–119

Further reading

Highlighted are three texts which will assist the reader in exploring the issues of ageism and the law.

Ashton G R 1995 Elderly people and the law. Butterworth, London
This is a text that specifically relates to the law and elderly people. Apart from its theoretical framework it offers the public as well as managers practical examples in areas such as care contracts, the drawing up of a will and enduring power of attorney.

Redfern S, Ross F 1999 Nursing older people, 3rd edn. Churchill Livingstone, Edinburgh
This is a comprehensive text that examines interprofessional working and challenges policy.

Wade L, Waters K R 1995 A textbook of gerontological nursing. Baillière Tindall, London
This takes a holistic approach towards older people, challenging many ageist assumptions. Personal testimonies from providers of care and those living within the community challenge both societal and professional prejudices.

Ageism and the law

Application **7:1**

Martin Johnston

Priority or prejudice?

INTRODUCTION

As has been evident throughout this book, a central feature of judging the effectiveness of service providers in meeting the needs of particular groups is related to access to services. Whether intentional or not, particular practices can be seen to lead to exclusion of particular groups. Consequently it is of paramount importance that we give very careful consideration to decisions regarding resource allocation and prioritising access to treatment.

The immediate tendency in health care is to consider apparently quantitative factors such as clinical need in the hope of avoiding unfairly biased value judgements. However, when faced with finite resources, clinical need alone may not enable us to decide between competing claims; it is not uncommon to encounter situations where clinical need is broadly equivalent. What becomes vital here is consideration of the possible influence of non-clinical factors and whether or not such factors are legitimate as a foundation for resource allocation decisions. The surprising feature is the distinct lack of empirical work looking at factors which influence attitudes towards resource allocation amongst service users.

One exception to this is the study by Mariotto et al (1999) concerning attitudes towards prioritisation of access to cardiac services. We shall consider this study in more detail as an example of how such research may be undertaken and as a contribution to the debate on resource allocation in its own right.

THE STUDY

The study concerned attitudes towards factors of age and employment status as grounds for prioritising access to cardiac services. Two groups were interviewed: a sample of elderly residents in the town of Padova, Italy, and a sample of nurses and nurses' aides, all of whom were involved in the care of the elderly. Respondents were presented with four scenarios and asked whether they thought it would be right to give up their place in a waiting list for another patient. Scenario 1 concerned allowing a younger patient to receive cardiac surgery and scenario 2 earlier attendance at an outpatients clinic. Scenarios 3 and 4 related to the same treatments but in this case the individual to benefit was self-employed. The results showed that in this hypothetical situation the elderly respondents were much more likely to think it right to give up their place in the queue in preference both to someone younger and to someone who was self-employed than the younger health care professionals, who were asked to imagine themselves as elderly. In the case of a younger patient awaiting cardiac surgery, 51% of the elderly sample were prepared to give up their place, with 68% agreeing to do so for the outpatient appointment and in the case of the self-employed patient, the figures were 47% and 68% for surgery and outpatient appointments respectively. The figures for the health professionals in each of the four cases were: 24%, 25%, 18% and 29%.

DISCUSSION

Now as with any research results, a degree of caution is required in generalising from a limited set of data and Mariotto et al (1999, p 469) are well aware of the limitations of their study. Nonetheless, there remains the interesting prima facie difference between elderly and younger respondents which requires some sort of explanation. We appear to have a group who are far more altruistic than their younger counterparts. That the explanation of this difference is complex is a point noted by the researchers who consider a range of factors like level of education, marital status and so on without any completely clear factor emerging, but it is to their credit that they make the attempt to explore the possibilities. But even in the absence of such clearly identified factors, it is still worthwhile to consider some possible explanations of the difference.

A point worth noting is the way the question was worded, with respondents being asked whether they thought it was right to give up a place. Quite clearly, there is something inherently ethical in this. What we see is that the elderly respondents appear more likely to include age as a factor which should be taken into account when prioritisation decisions are being taken, with the advantage going to younger patients and those who are self-employed. That there is a difference at all between the elderly respondents and health professionals should remind us of the variability of value judgements and the dangers of assuming that we can apply some universal system, and merits further investigation.

An interesting possibility raised by Mariotto et al (1999, p 470) themselves is that what we are witnessing is the internalisation of discriminatory attitudes towards the elderly, by the respondents. Factors such as loss of self-esteem and feelings of worthlessness may contribute to some elderly respondents feeling that it is their duty to stand aside in favour of the younger or apparently more productive but what is open to question is the validity of such judgements. What is the basis for presuming that younger or self-employed people are more useful or deserving? Unless we can provide some kind of definitive answer here, then we are dealing with prejudice and not rational prioritisation.

This point becomes all the more significant when we consider the broader context of health care provision for the elderly. Phair (1999) highlights the difficulties associated with long-term care, where apparently innocuous decisions about whether a home be registered as 'nursing' or 'residential' can have profound implications for both the quality and cost of care to an elderly client. Taking a yet broader perspective, Parker (1999) highlights the apparent failure of the Royal Commission on Long-Term Care to meet its own expressed objective to promote debate concerning long-term care. All of which points to a reluctance to address issues relating to health care provision and the elderly in anything like a direct and open manner.

CONCLUSION

What this brief review of research and literature suggests is the need for much more extensive work. The work of Mariotto et al (1999) provides a useful starting point for identifying the values which underpin individual choices and is applicable in a variety of contexts. Similarly, the rigour with which they undertake the analysis of their results provides a foundation for further study. It is only through such detailed inquiry that we can hope to provide rational and legitimate foundations for the difficult decisions regarding resource allocation and prioritisation of treatment which confront contemporary health services. A failure to do so shifts our decision making dangerously down the path of prejudice.

References

Mariotto A, De Leo D, Buono M D, Favaretti C, Austin P, Naylor C D 1999 Will elderly patients stand aside for younger patients in the queue for cardiac services? Lancet 354:467–470

Parker G 1999 Long-term care for older people: the unanswered questions. Journal of Health Service Research Policy 4:131–132

Phair L 1999 Inequality in care for older people. Nursing Management 6:14–17

MANAGING CHANGE: DIVERSITY, THE KEY TO SUCCESS

Chapter **Eight**

Diversity, change and the professional manager

Steve Willcocks

OVERVIEW

The purpose of this chapter is to introduce the reader to recent organisational change theory and practice and discuss the relevance of this to NHS organisations which are employers of people from, and delivers services to, a diverse population. It begins with an overview of the context of diversity, particularly the policy changes of the 1980s and 1990s, and discusses the extent to which these changes represent incremental or transformational change.

Then follows an introduction to organisational change theory and a selective review of some key influential approaches, specifically: organisation development, the contextualist approach to change, including political and cultural views, and the contribution of learning theory and the concept of the learning organisation. We attempt to assess the significance of these specific approaches for managers and nurses who are managing change in the NHS but conclude that no one approach is right: that a pluralistic and diverse organisation such as the NHS may need to be eclectic in its use of approaches.

Objectives

This chapter explores the following themes and issues:

- the policy context and background of managerial changes in the NHS
- the idea of incremental and transformational change
- approaches to organisational change, theory and problems
- some specific approaches:
  - organisation development (OD) and its relevance to nurses and health care management
  - contextualist approaches to change: the importance of cultural and political aspects of change in the context of diversity
  - learning theory and change: individual learning, organisational learning and 'the learning organisation' in the NHS.

CHANGE IN THE NHS: THE POLICY CONTEXT

Introduction

One of the most significant policy changes in the 1980s and 1990s was the introduction of managerialism in the public sector. Observers have debated the extent to which this has represented a challenge to traditional administrative and professional cultures which were historically dominant in the sector. For some, managerialism represented a shift in the management of the public sector, from old-style 'public administration' to new forms, collectively known as 'new public management' (Gunn 1989, p 21).

It has been suggested that the changes involved a major shift or redistribution of power in the public sector, from dominant professionals to the new public sector managers, with the possible ascendancy of entrepreneurial values in contrast to traditional professional values (Ferlie 1994) although this has been disputed (for example, Hunter 1994, p 21). Ferlie (1994) has characterised 'new public management' as the dominant form in the 1980s and early 1990s, underpinned by 'value for money', concern for efficiency and strong management, an increased responsiveness to consumers and a more entrepreneurial management style. This had considerable impact on nursing staff and nurse managers, in terms of changing expectations about their role and contribution to the NHS.

The Griffiths reforms in the NHS

The earliest expression of this form of managerialism in the NHS was the policy resulting from the Griffiths Inquiry (DoH 1983). Griffiths, a private sector business manager, presented a detailed diagnosis of the problems of managing the NHS: there was a lack of strategic direction; a failure to identify individual managerial responsibility (based partly on a critique of the consensus management teams introduced in 1974); a lack of focus on objectives and performance; and little orientation towards the 'consumer' of the service (Harrison et al 1988, pp 27–28). The Griffiths Inquiry resulted in the introduction of general management into the health service; the idea was to 'create a more proactive vision of management, to create a new managerial cadre' (Harrison & Pollitt 1994, p 39), with an expectation that general managers would be agents of change.

The Griffiths reforms heralded the start of a series of initiatives aimed at strengthening the management arrangements in the service. They were, however, essentially changes to the existing structural configuration of the NHS and had a particular impact upon the hitherto dominant hierarchical management approach in nursing. They continued up to the late 1980s, by which time a more fundamental and radical review of the health service was under way, prompted by continuing political concern about the need to improve efficiency and management.

The reforms of 1990

The new ideas emanating from the White Paper '*Working for patients*' (DoH 1989) and subsequently introduced in the NHS and Community Care Act 1990 were partly a further extension or reinforcement of managerialism in the health service. However, compared to earlier reforms, it has been suggested (Ashburner et al 1996) that they represented a more radical or transformational change, particularly the introduction of competition by a 'quasi-market' or internal market in health care and the separation of the NHS into purchasing and providing authorities. In addition to this general objective, there was also emphasis upon the need to involve professionals in the running of the service and following on from these reforms, professionals (particularly doctors) were incorporated into decentralised management structures. The latter introduced new lines of managerial accountability for nursing staff. In the hospital sector, new managerial teams headed by

Diversity, change and the professional manager

clinical directors were expected to manage clinical services and plan and initiate change in service delivery. There was thus a continuing emphasis on the ability to introduce and implement change by conscious managerial action. Clinical directors, alongside nurse and business managers, were expected to take the lead and be proactive in implementing the change agenda.

In the primary care sector, innovation in purchasing created a new organisational form, GP fundholding, and for some observers (for example, Glennerster et al 1994) this was considered a qualified success. In particular, GP fundholders were said to have helped shift the balance of power in medicine away from hospitals, provided greater consumer focus (for fundholding patients) and become a force for change in service delivery.

The reforms of 1997

These reforms, in turn, were followed by numerous developments in the 1990s, with a progressive shift away from secondary to primary care led-service and a concern for improving management in the latter.

In 1997, with a change of government, a new White Paper, *The new NHS: modern, dependable* (DoH 1997), heralded another major reform programme for the health service and a whole series of further changes. While this announced the end of competition and the internal market and an intention to remedy perceived problems such as fragmentation and inequity in service provision, there is a strong element of continuity in the attempt to improve management of the service. The reforms continued to emphasise efficiency, performance monitoring, the use of national standards and guidelines and national frameworks reminiscent of the Griffiths Inquiry.

However, there was also a recognition of the need to address a perceived overemphasis on efficiency by bringing quality and efficiency closer together and putting further emphasis on introducing an evidence-based approach to health care. At local level, nurses and other professionals working in primary and secondary care are required to develop and implement a new system of clinical governance, with the intention of improving the quality of clinical care.

In primary care, a new organisation, the primary care group (PCG) has been created to replace previous innovations such as fundholding, total purchasing pilots and locality commissioning groups. PCGs will be involved in both operational and strategic management and may have both commissioning and providing functions. The management boards for these organisations, and particularly for the primary care trusts which may emerge, provide new managerial challenges for general practitioners, nurses and other professionals.

In all, the reforms of 1997 and subsequent policy guidelines from the Department of Health represent opportunities as well as challenges for nurses and nurse managers. Nurses will need to reconsider the values, beliefs and assumptions underpinning further change; for example, they may need to reconsider the extent to which this further development of managerialism is compatible with and capable of delivering the change agenda and the extent to which it will provide for greater equality, equity, diversity and consumer involvement in service delivery.

These represent important cultural and political aspects of change which will inevitably be crucial to the success or otherwise of the latest reform programme. Nurses and other professionals need a good understanding of organisational change theory and practice in order to ensure that these and other issues are fully considered and accounted for.

UNDERSTANDING ORGANISATIONAL CHANGE

Incremental or radical change?

This section begins to map out some ideas about organisational change and will subsequently examine particular approaches which might be relevant to nurses. Hitherto, change in the NHS has been said to fit more closely with the notion of 'first-order' change or incremental change (Ashburner et al 1996). Since the beginning of the 1990s attempts to introduce politically driven top-down change in the NHS can be said to be 'radical' change in which: 'the organisation is required to move from known and established behavioural patterns to new behaviours of which the organisation has no real experience' (Todd 1999). This type of change 'invariably touches on the core purpose of the organisation' (Benjamin & Mabey 1993) and thus is intimately concerned with attempting to change the culture of the NHS.

This distinction between incremental or 'first-order' change and radical or 'second-order' change may serve as a guide to nursing staff and managers in selecting an appropriate change approach (Table 8.1).

Diversity, change and the professional manager

Managing change: diversity, the key to success

> **Table 8.1** Change approaches (based on State 1996, p 559)
>
> | Change type | Change approach | Emphasis |
> |---|---|---|
> | Developmental transitions | Organisation development (OD) – US | Incremental change, derived from human relations: deliberative, involving people |
> | | Japanese management | Involving workforce in shopfloor management and process improvement |
> | Task-focused transitions | Sociotechnical change – UK Tavistock tradition | Emphasis on changing the system, involving workforce |
> | Charismatic transformation | Organisation transformation (OT) – US | Revolutionary (radical) change, led by visionary inspiring leader |
> | Turnaround | Pragmatic, economic, rationalism, pluralistic | Revolutionary change, decisive, coercive |

Approaches to organisational change

This section will review some approaches to organisational change although, given the variety of approaches, this will inevitably be selective. The first problem in writing about organisational change is the fact that there is little agreement or consensus about theory and practice-based approaches. It has been argued that the literature on organisational change is fragmented (Buchanan & Badham 1999) and that there is no generally accepted theory about organisational change (Dunphy 1996). The latter has suggested that a fully fledged theory of change should embrace the following elements:

- a basic metaphor of the organisation – a descriptive summary
- an analytical framework or diagnostic model
- an 'ideal' model of an effectively functioning organisation
- an intervention theory
- a definition of the role of the change agent (Dunphy 1996, p 543).

These elements are suggested as a way of comparing the advantages and disadvantages of different approaches to organisational change. They also recognise the need to build a bridge between theoretical and practice-based approaches and between 'ideal' models and reality. For professionals such as nursing staff, this is a particularly relevant consideration.

One problem with approaches to organisational change is the distinction between prescriptive, 'one best way' approaches, management 'recipes' (Wilson 1992) or 'cook books' (Spurgeon & Barwell 1991) and theoretically driven approaches with a focus on the analysis of organisational change. Wilson (1992) warns us to be wary of 'models' of change:

> Upon what intellectual basis (or bases) are models of change constructed? What are the assumptions and what are the prevailing theories in use? What are the definitions of change that are used? What is the degree of supporting empirical evidence? (Wilson 1992, p 8)

The problem is compounded by the fact that these two approaches – prescriptive and descriptive – are not necessarily compatible; hence, 'there is a gulf between theory and practice which requires bridging' (Spurgeon & Barwell 1991, pp 34–35). However, there is a popular appeal to managers in prescriptive 'off-the-shelf' solutions to managing organisational change. Some of the prescriptive approaches to change have become the dominant ideology, particularly organisation development (OD) and, more recently, the idea of the 'heroic' entrepreneur, the charismatic leader of planned organisational change (Peters & Waterman 1982).

SOME SPECIFIC APPROACHES

Chronologically, the literature on change stretches way back into the 1960s and before. Most textbooks on organisational change would probably highlight the emergence of OD in the United States and sociotechnical systems, based on the work of researchers at the Tavistock Institute in the UK. The latter approach utilises systems thinking as an analytical framework for managing change and is still influential (see McCalman & Paton 1992, p 49). The former has had a long history and was dominant until recently, although it is said to remain of contemporary relevance:

> The action research model, a systems approach to understanding organisational dynamics and a change strategy that focuses on the

Diversity, change and the professional manager

culture of work teams and the organisation – all these features of organisation development serve to make it more powerful and relevant than most change strategies of the past. (Mukherji & Mukherji 1998, p 269)

Organisation development

Organisation development (OD) is said to be a prescriptive approach to planned organisational change (Spurgeon & Barwell 1991). It aims to be: 'a long-term strategic mechanism for initiating change which places emphasis on the process of attaining change' (McCalman & Paton 1992, p 134).

The overriding principle is 'an ideology of participative incrementalism' (Stace 1996, p 555), a view that sees 'change as best taking place incrementally, on the basis of consensus, collaboration and participation' (Quinn, in Ashburner et al 1996). French & Bell (1973) provide an often-quoted definition of the approach:

> Organisation development is a top management supported, long-range effort to improve an organisation's problem-solving and renewal processes, particularly through a more effective and collaborative diagnosis and management of organisation culture – with special emphasis on formal work team, temporary team and intergroup culture. (French & Bell 1973, p 17)

This definition emphasises the importance of collaborative problem solving and renewal; its advocacy of action research as a methodology to facilitate this is said to be one of its strengths. It also focuses specifically upon the team and this is particularly relevant to nurses and nurse managers working in the NHS.

The theory underpinning OD was provided by Lewin (1951). This focuses upon a three-stage 'pattern' or process, beginning with unfreezing (present behaviour), then movement (taking action) and refreezing of new behaviour. A more recent but similar version is provided by Schein (1987).

1. *Unfreezing* – creating motivation and readiness for change by disconfirmation, induction of anxiety or guilt or creation of psychological safety.
2. *Changing or cognitive restructuring* – movement.
3. *Refreezing* – integrating the change process through personal refreezing and relational refreezing, and integrating with others.

It has been suggested that most accounts of organisational change implicitly follow this pattern (Hendry 1996, p 624). However, it does raise the question whether the change process really is quite

Managing change: diversity, the key to success

so straightforward, sequential and logical and do nurses and health care managers really possess the knowledge and skills to manage change in this way?

Another well-known OD conceptualisation is provided by Beckhard & Harris (1987). This is also centred upon a three-stage process of change.

1. *The present state* – dissatisfaction with the present. Where are we now (for example, in terms of implementing evidence-based practice in nursing)?
2. *The desired future state* – identify goals – where do we want to be (for example, practice informed by the latest research evidence)?
3. *Transition state* – movement from 1 to 2 – how do we get there (what specific actions are needed to facilitate this change?)?

The advantage of this perspective on change is that it provides a framework within which to evaluate present and future goals, policies and priorities and an emphasis on the implementation phase. Beckhard & Harris argue for the importance of effective management of the transition stage; in other words, managing the transition from present to desired future state and minimising personal and organisational disruption. This is important for any manager or nursing professional aiming to introduce change in practice or organisation.

The collaborative and processual basis of OD may be particularly relevant in the nursing context, given the action research-based emphasis, involving professionals and users in managing service delivery. The emphasis on process may also be appropriate: there has been a tendency to neglect process and implementation issues in successive health care reorganisations and major changes and in particular, to neglect the role that nurses will have to play within this process.

The notion of an 'unfreezing' phase in the change process directs attention to the learning and unlearning that may need to take place in order to facilitate transformational or even incremental change. This may particularly apply to professionals working in the NHS; for example, nurses in primary care, faced with the prospect of considerable upheaval or disturbance, resulting from the 1997 reforms in the primary care sector. It may apply at the organisational or practice level; for example, it may be relevant to nurses attempting to change practice, introduce evidence-based care, clinical governance and so forth.

However, OD has been criticised for paying insufficient attention to the wider historical, economic and political context

Diversity, change and the professional manager

of change (Wilson 1992). Furthermore, it has been criticised because of its inability to comprehend notions of transformatory or second-order change (Ashburner et al 1996); for example:

> The OD tradition, lacking a contextual or environmental element, had difficulty explaining the rise of coercive reorganisations apparent in the 1980s, often introduced by the dictate of newly imposed chief executives. (Ashburner et al 1996, p 2)

OD has also been criticised for its neglect of organisational politics and issues of power (Buchanan & Badham 1999), for its adoption of highly rational and linear views of process (Pettigrew 1985) and for its emphasis on the social (people) system at the expense of task, technical, structure and strategy (Mukherji & Mukherji 1998). It has been considered more an 'ideal' than 'realised' model (Stace 1996).

The latter suggests that many theorists have moved sideways to develop a variation of OD: organisation transformation (OT) but with a similar concern for collaboration or consultation, and with emphasis upon charismatic leadership (Stace 1996, pp 559–560). Similarly, Stace believes that the popularity of Japanese management techniques in the late 1980s was partly because of the links with OD but questions the cultural specificity of the Japanese model (Stace 1996, p 560).

For staff working in the NHS, particularly nursing staff, the neglect of historical, cultural and political factors related to organisational change is a potentially serious omission.

Contextual approach to change

These criticisms of OD have partly emerged from the work of theorists offering an empirically derived perspective on the management of change. The 'contextualist' approach is associated with the work at Warwick (for example, Pettigrew 1985, Pettigrew et al 1992). The emphasis is on an 'expanded focus': 'not only processual factors but also the historical, cultural and political features of organisational change' (Spurgeon & Barwell 1991) or, in other words, the context of change. It is necessary to acknowledge the interplay between *context* of change, the *process* of change and the *content* of change. Success in managing change is 'highly contextually sensitive, suggesting that "off the shelf" solutions and individual competencies may have only limited and partial impact' (Pettigrew et al 1992, p 27). This approach defines change management as a: 'jointly analytical, educational/learning, and political process' (Pettigrew & Whipp, 1991) and is in contrast to rational, planned approaches to organisational change. The latter is said to

Managing change: diversity, the key to success

ignore the context of change and implicitly advocates: 'uncritical acceptance of the manager as both agent and sole determinant of organisational change' (Wilson 1992, p 12).

This approach may offer an alternative focus for nurses seeking to ensure that organisational change takes account of, or addresses, issues of diversity relating to gender, age, race, culture and so forth.

The emphasis on understanding the context of this is particularly seen in the notion of receptive and non-receptive contexts for change; the idea that there are 'signs and symptoms of receptivity to change in an organisation', consisting of eight features:

- environmental pressure to change; for example, politically driven pressure
- the quality and coherence of policy, nationally from the centre and locally
- key people leading the change, a critical mass of change supporters
- effective managerial/clinical relations are seen as crucial in the NHS
- cooperative interorganisation networks, particularly relevant in the post-1997 NHS
- simplicity and clarity of goals
- the change agenda and its locale, ensuring a 'good fit'
- supportive organisational culture – another crucial under-pinning to any change programme (Pettigrew et al 1992, p 29).

The presence of these eight factors, which are seen as dynamic, changing and capable of influence, is said to provide a 'linked set of conditions which provide high energy around change' (Pettigrew et al 1992, p 28). Nurses and other staff may find these particularly relevant to the analysis of change in the NHS and, indeed, they have been applied to the NHS by these authors. They reinforce the importance of understanding change in the NHS by analysis of specific contexts and through understanding of process. This approach also draws attention to the importance of political and cultural factors in these contexts; for example, the culture context in the NHS may be resistant to change. Hendry (1996) has pointed out that the most difficult aspect of change is getting started; this goes beyond changing cognitive structures and embraces cultural change, change in basic assumptions, values and beliefs. This can be facilitated by political intervention or by attempting to influence organisational culture: both approaches share a concern for *legitimation* (Hendry 1996); ideas can be legitimated and meanings managed.

Diversity, change and the professional manager

A radical top-down version of this emerged with Peters & Waterman (1982) and other US writers:

> They recommend starting by changing the organisational artefacts such as mission, vision, or core value statement and then align the behaviour of all parts of the organisation behind these. (Hawkins 1997, p 432)

The latter author labels this the heroic school of management development, the impact of the charismatic leader on changing organisational culture. The problem with this view is that it assumes a passive subordinated role for members of the organisation such as nursing staff in a hospital and a view of culture as 'owned' or manipulated by management. This may also be consistent with the view of nurses who may feel alienated from 'management'.

A problem with the contextualist view is that it fails to take account of the fact that specific contexts may be 'enacted' (Weick 1979), comprising what people give attention to and how they interpret them (Hendry 1996, p 626).

However, an understanding or 'diagnosis' of the political and cultural context of change seems particularly relevant to the NHS. It is important for professionals and nurses involved in change to understand the dynamics of particular contexts and the interplay of historical, political, socioeconomic and cultural factors. This was important, for example, in a study of the implementation of managed competition in the NHS (Ranade 1995). The importance of the situation or context in organisational change is emphasised by Stace: 'best practice is eclectic, pragmatic, and culturally and situationally attuned' (Stace 1996, p 566). This is particularly relevant to and consistent with approaches to managing diversity.

Learning theory and change

Hendry has commented that the 'management of change literature has come to be characterised by a theoretical pragmatism, and, in reaction to previous neglect, it has arguably overfocused on the political aspects of the change process' (Hendry 1996, p 621). He attempts to remedy this by developing an approach to change which takes account of learning concepts. He argues that learning theory should be more central within planned organisational change.

This leads us to currently popular work on the concept of the 'learning organisation'. This emerged in the late 1980s with Hayes et al (1988) in the USA and Pedler et al (1988) in the UK but it can trace links or similarities with, for example, OD, action research, systems thinking and learning theory. The idea of a 'learning organisation' (say, an NHS trust hospital) is that it: 'facilitates the learning of all its members and continuously transforms itself' (Pedler et al 1988).

In more detail, a learning organisation:

> has a climate in which individual members are encouraged to learn and develop their full potential; extends this learning culture to include 'customers', suppliers and other significant stakeholders; values human resource development strategy central to business policy; is in a continuous process of organisational transformation. (Woodall & Winstanley 1998, p 150)

The application of these concepts to organisational transformation or change is said to be: 'one response to the increasing organisational challenges posed by rapid environmental change, discontinuity, uncertainty, complexity and globalisation' (Altman & Iles 1998, p 44).

There is a link to the contextualist approach: for example, Jones & Hendry (1994) suggest the need for more research to reveal the type of contexts that encourage learning and enable an organisation to change and transform in this way. This is important in relation to nurses in the NHS: for example, there may be relevance in viewing the new PCGs as emerging or developing learning organisations. It may be relevant to establish how individual learning by nurses and organisational learning and transformation may be facilitated and how this relates to other professionals, particularly general practitioners.

In this context, learning is both individual and organisational. The latter is not simply *'adaptive'* learning (about coping with change) but *'generative'* learning 'which is about creating new ways of looking at the world' (Senge 1990). This is similar to the concept of 'single and double loop' learning, the former questioning how things are done, the latter questioning why things are done (Altman & Iles 1998). The latter may be particularly relevant in nursing staff, given the current emphasis on research or evidence-based practice, and it also has strong links with the principles underpinning the introduction of clinical governance. There is also a link with Lewinian concepts of organisational change (Hendry 1996). For example, the latter points out that change as a learning process is apparent in Lewin's 'unfreezing' stage in the change management process. He suggests that:

> The kinds of problems that organisations encounter during change can be described, then, in learning terms, while a learning organisation is one that tries to model itself round lessons from change. (Hendry 1996, p 629)

It has to be said that learning may also be a barrier to or inhibitor of change and one of the requirements may be 'undoing' prior learning or using disconformation as a way of stimulating change. This may also be relevant to change in the NHS, particularly in relation to possible nurse or professional resistance to change. In other words, learning may be a force for inertia as well as a dynamic of change.

Another important strand of learning theory is the attempt to integrate individual and organisational learning. Altman & Iles (1998) attempt to integrate these concepts through the development of a model which advocates leadership and teams as the key transformative processes. Similarly, Hendry (1996) proposes the idea of 'communities of practice' (relationships formed to solve problems) which engage in learning from experience, develop cognitive structures and facilitate cultural change. Both ideas may be relevant to nurses in the NHS: in recent years there has been a renewed interest in the concept of the integrated team (for example, the multidisciplinary clinical team) and in how these teams may be able to facilitate learning and change.

In general, the learning approach to change provides a useful focus for knowledge-based organisations like the NHS. In order to facilitate learning, nurses and nurse managers need to debate answers to the following questions.

- What is learning in the context of nursing practice?
- How does the organisation facilitate and inhibit learning for nurses?
- What is it that is transformed, and when, where, why?
- As an organisation and individual nurses are transformed, does this process occur at one time?
- Is that which is being transformed a processual or instant activity?
- Is the idea of 'transformation' misleading?
- Do we mean simply adapting and changing when the word 'transform' is used?
- What drives the transformation process? (based on Jones & Hendry 1994, p 155)

CONCLUSION

This chapter has examined the policy context of change in the NHS. It has followed this with a critical review of organisational change theory and practice, recognising that this remains subject to debate and lack of agreement, with little consensus on the way forward. Given the enormous range of work on organisational change, it has been highly selective in its review of specific approaches. It has attempted to examine the strengths and weaknesses of three specific approaches: organisation development (OD); the contextualist approach; and the concept of the learning organisation and change. It has found that while they each have limitations, they also provide some insight for nurses and other professionals who need to understand organisational change in the NHS. It can be argued that, given the pluralistic and diverse nature of the NHS, an eclectic and pragmatic approach to managing change is required.

It has been shown that OD may be useful for nurses and professionals, in terms of serving a collaborative purpose (a policy priority in the NHS) via its advocacy of action research methodology. It also serves to remind NHS managers, nurses and other professionals of the importance of the *process* of change, not just the *content*, as has been the case in the past. It also suggests that to be successful, change must take account of the need to 'unfreeze' existing patterns of behaviour, habit and working practices. (However, for professionals and nurses to successfully manage the process of change, it requires management development of an order which has never occurred before.)

The contextualist approach has pointed to the importance of understanding the change context, particularly the historical, cultural and political context in the NHS. This is seen as absent or underplayed in OD but in terms of the NHS this context is vital.

The final approach – learning theory and the learning organisation – offers a corrective to the recent overemphasis on the political factors and argues for the utility of learning concepts as an aid to understanding change. This approach is useful to the nurses and professionals because it shows the importance of interrelated, individual and organisational learning underpinning change programmes and the fact that specific contexts may inhibit or support such learning and there is a need to break down such barriers if managing diversity is to become a positive strength in the NHS. The idea of the learning organisation may be applied to NHS organisations (lifelong learning and continuing professional

Diversity, change and the professional manager

development are key themes in the 1997 White Paper), particularly organisations about to transform themselves, and learning theory is relevant to individuals involved in such transformations, particularly professionals.

Practice checklist

Readers should consider the following issues which may inform practice.

- The importance of understanding the *context* of change and its interrelationships with *content* of change and *process* of change (Pettigrew et al 1992).
- The multidimensional character of organisational change and the insights made possible by examining it through different perspectives.
- The relevance of particular approaches to organisational change to their own practice/context, recognising that there is 'no one right way'.
- The importance of recognising the lifelong learning required in order to maintain organisational and professional integrity in the face of organisational change.

Discussion questions

- As a manager or nurse, you are invited to reflect upon your recent experience in managing or being part of a specific change in your organisation/unit.
  - To what extent did this change recognise and reflect the specific cultural and political context?
  - Did the change plan pay adequate attention to the *process* of introducing change and if not, why not?
- Comment upon your preferred approach to managing organisational change and why you feel it is particularly appropriate to your own context.
- Identify and discuss your personal learning requirements which might be necessary to prepare you for the latest changes being introduced by the White Paper *The new NHS: modern, dependable* (DoH 1997).

References

Altman Y, Iles P 1998 Learning, leadership, teams: corporate learning and organisational change. Journal of Management 17(1):44–55

Managing change: diversity, the key to success

Ashburner L, Ferlie E, Fitzgerald L 1996 Organisational transformation and top down change: the case of the NHS. British Journal of Management 7(1):1–16

Beckhard R, Harris R T 1987 Organisational transitions: managing complex change. Addison-Wesley, Reading, MA

Benjamin G, Mabey C 1993 Facilitating radical change: a case of organisation transformation. In: Mabey C, Mayon-White B (eds) Managing change. Paul Chapman, London

Buchanan D, Badham R 1999 Politics and organisational change: the lived experience. Human Relations 52(5):609–629

Department of Health 1983 NHS management enquiry (Griffiths Report). HMSO, London

Department of Health 1989 Working for patients. HMSO, London

Department of Health 1997 The new NHS: modern, dependable. Stationery Office, London

Dunphy D 1996 Organisational change in corporate settings. Human Relations 49 (5):541–551

Ferlie E 1994 Characterising the new public management. Paper presented at the Annual Conference of the British Acadamy of Management, September, pp 12–14

French W L, Bell C H 1973 Organisation development: behavioural science intervention for organisation improvement. Prentice Hall, Englewood Cliffs, NJ

Glennerster H, Matsaganis M, Owens P 1994 Implementing GP fundholding. Open University Press, Buckingham

Gunn L 1989 A public management approach to the NHS. Health Service Management Research 2(1):10–91

Harrison S, Pollitt C 1994 Controlling health professionals: the future of work and organisation in the NHS. Open University Press, Buckingham

Harrison S, Hunter D J, Marnoch G, Politt C 1988 Check out on Griffiths: general management in the NHS. ESRC Newsletter 62:27–28

Hawkins P 1997 Organisation culture: sailing between evangelism and complexity. Human Relations 50(4):417–440

Hayes R H, Wheelwright S C, Clark K B 1988 Dynamics manufacturing: creating the learning organisation. Free Press, New York

Hendry C 1996 Understanding and creating whole organisational change through learning theory. Human Relations 49(5):621–641

Hunter D J 1994 From tribalism to corporatism: the managerial challenge to the medical dominance. In: Gabe J, Kelleher D, Williams E (eds) Challenging medicine. Routledge, London

Jones A M, Hendry C 1994 The learning organisation: adult learning and organisational transformation. British Journal of Management 5:153–162

Lewin K 1951 Field theory in social science. Harper and Row, New York

McCalman J, Paton R A 1992 Change management: a guide to effective implementation. Paul Chapman, London

Mukherji A, Mukherji J 1998 Structuring organisations for the future: analysing and managing change. Management Decision 36(4):265–273

Diversity, change and the professional manager

Pedler M, Boydell T, Burgoyne J 1988 Learning company project: a report on work undertaken Oct 1987 – April 1989. Training Agency, Sheffield

Peters T J, Waterman R H 1982 In search of excellence. Harper and Row, New York

Pettigrew A M 1985 The awakening giant. Blackwell, Oxford

Pettigrew A M, Whipp R 1991 Managing change for competitive success. Blackwell, Oxford

Pettigrew A M, Ferlie E, McKee L 1992 Shaping strategic change: the case of the NHS in the 1980's. Public Money and Management 27–31

Ranade W 1995 The theory and practice of managed competition in the NHS. Public Administration 73:241–262

Schein E H 1987 Process consultation vol 2: lessons for managers and consultants. Addison-Wesley, Reading, MA

Senge P 1990 The leaders new work: building learning organisations. Sloan Management Review Fall: 7–22

Spurgeon P, Barwell F 1991 Implementing change in the NHS. Chapman and Hall, London

Stace D A 1996 Dominant ideologies, strategic change and sustained performance. Human Relations 149(5):551–570

Todd A 1999 Managing radical change. Long Range Planning 32(2):237–244

Weick K E 1979 The social psychology of organising. Addison-Wesley, Reading, MA

Wilson D 1992 A strategy of change. Routledge, London

Woodall J, Winstanley D 1998 Management development: strategy and practice. Blackwell, Oxford

Further reading

Ferlie E, Pettigrew A, Ashburner L, Fitzgerald L 1996 The new public management in action. Oxford University Press, Oxford

Mabey C, Mayon-White B (eds) 1993 Managing change. Paul Chapman, London

McCalman J, Paton R A 1992 Change management: a guide to effective implementation. Paul Chapman, London

Spurgeon P, Barwell F 1991 Implementing change in the NHS; a practical guide for general managers. Chapman and Hall, London

Managing change: diversity, the key to success

Chapter Nine

The cultural competence model

Barbara Burford

OVERVIEW

If we are to develop professionals who are competent in today's multicultural milieux then it is essential that we address a number of key elements. This chapter thus presents an expressing of these elements and offers a brief overview and discussion of the literature on culture and competence. Further, it explores the concepts and models of cultural competency current in the UK and USA and examines their relevance in today's environment.

INTRODUCTION

At present both the word 'culture' and, to a lesser extent, the word 'competence' have become part of 'business speak' and their separate meanings have become labile in the extreme. Most business theorists and writers, from Fayol to Taylor to Moss Kanter, comment on and agree that the culture of the organisation is a primary variable in that entity's ability to deliver its strategic objectives. Whole curricula and indeed mini-industries have been built on issues of organisational and business culture and how to survive, change or develop it or indeed how to teach any or all of these things. We have seen the culture of an organisation described as 'X' – directive with an innate suspicion of the worker commitment to the task – or 'Y' – with an interest in the personal and relationship needs of the workers – by McGregor in the 1960s and then again as 'Z', in his examinations of how America could learn from the Japanese, by Ouchi in the 1980s. Major theorists and writers on strategy such as Porter, Beckhard, Waterman and Minzberg have all maintained the importance of being able to analyse the current culture of an enterprise and to prescribe the culture required to deliver new objectives as well as the levers within an organisation that enable and aid the shift in culture.

This chapter briefly reviews the literature on culture and competence, then moves to a detailed analysis of the published work on cultural competence, both in the USA and in the UK.

WHAT DOES CULTURE MEAN IN THIS CONTEXT?

Culture, in the business sense and at its simplest and most familiar definition, is about 'the way we do things round here' (Bower 1966). This view sees the organisation acting as its own mini-world with a set of intrinsic values and an emotional and reward currency that is perhaps unique to that sector or even that organisation.

In its older senses, culture could mean anthropologically either the great or quaint civilisations of the past. The value judgements are dependent upon those of the culture from which these others are viewed. So, conceivably, one of the variables of culture could be perspective. Culture can also mean the same as 'civilised', again a question of perspective. Beckhard & Harris (1987) make an important distinction between the *culture* of an organisation and its *climate*. They write that while the climate of the organisation is the 'measure of the morale or happiness of the staff at any particular time. What we mean by culture is a set of artifacts, beliefs, values, norms, and ground rules that defines and significantly influences how the organisation operates'. There is also the view expressed by Minzberg (1983), amongst others, that although organisational culture is inanimate, it often seems to have a self-perpetuating life of its own.

WHAT DOES COMPETENCE MEAN IN THIS CONTEXT?

Among the many dictionary definitions of competence are ability, capability, expertise, mastery, proficiency and skill. However, while there is surprisingly little in the business literature about competence, what there is is unexpectedly confused. There is a lack of clarity about the differences between competence, competencies and competency. Miller (1993), discussing the nature of strategic management, comments on Prahalad & Hamel's (1990) definition of 'core competences' as 'the collective learning in an organisation' and the 'communication, involvement, and … deep commitment to working across organisational boundaries'. She finds them unsatisfactorily vague about how this could be of practical use to an organisation. In her work on district nurse competencies, Young (1997) writes:

> …competence involves the mastery of requirements for effective functioning, in the varied circumstances of the real world, and in a range of contexts and organisations. It involves not only observable behaviour that can be measured, but also unobservable attributes including attitudes, values, judgemental ability and personal dispositions.

WHAT DOES 'CULTURAL COMPETENCE' MEAN?

If, as discussed in the introduction, organisational culture is a manifestation not just of the history and people of the organisation but also of the history and people of the nation in which the organisation is based (Hofstede 1980) and if, as Minzberg (1983) believes, organisational cultures can acquire 'a life of their own', how can we define cultural competence?

The cultural competence model

Leininger (1978) believed that transcultural nursing which showed cultural competence involved being able to provide care that was culturally specific but to also include those universal care practices which were appropriate. At the University of Texas Medical School, Thorpe & Baker (1995) described cultural competence as '... the ability to think and behave in ways that enable a member of one culture to work effectively with members of another culture'. While Wells (1995), of the American Occupational Therapy Association, describes cultural competence as '... accepting and understanding a variety of customs, values, beliefs ...', Campinha-Bacote (1994a) sees cultural competence as: '... a process in which the psychiatric-mental health nurse sees himself or herself always in the process of *becoming* culturally competent rather than *being* culturally competent'. She proposes a model of cultural competence in psychiatric nursing which includes cultural awareness, cultural knowledge, cultural skill and cultural encounters.

Gerrish et al (1996) propose a model for cultural competence which is made up initially of 'cultural communicative competence' which is about learning to '... understand the cultural values, behavioural patterns and rules for interaction in specific cultures'. The second part of the concept is 'intercultural communicative competence' and draws on the work of Kim (1992) which suggests that these are a generic set of skills which rely on the practitioner's learned ability to learn quickly what is important in communicating with a particular culture.

EVOLUTION AND DEVELOPMENT

The literature on cultural competence in nursing, particularly in psychiatric nursing, is largely from the USA where it grew out of the explicit espousal of the 'melting pot' theory of social and community evolution: '... for nearly one in three Americans will be a minority by the year 2000' (Campinha-Bacote 1994a). The attitude was that somehow, by acquiring the right behaviours, attitudes and aspirations or simply by espousing them until one has sworn citizenship, one could become an American. Later, influenced by Glynn & Rockarts (1986) and others, there was a shift from this concept. Because America and Americans were beginning to be seen as made up of different communities, appropriate provision had to be made in both private and state services to ensure equality of access and outcome.

As early as 1967 nurses and other health care educators such as Leininger were beginning to question the ability of practitioners to deliver care to a multiethnic population (Leininger 1967, 1978). Each writer built on or developed further models for the delivery of what Leininger called cultural specific care or later transcultural nursing. Early models spoke of 'ethnic-sensitive practice' (Devore & Schlesinger 1981), 'ethnic competence' (Green 1982) or 'ethnic minority practice' (Lum 1986). However, gradually the term 'culture' began to be substituted for 'ethnic' and the term 'cultural competence', although having many different definitions, became the shorthand for this whole field of effort: how to provide sensitive and appropriate care across barriers of language, upbringing, ethnicity and culture and in particular how to train practitioners to do so. In the late 1980s and early 1990s, there was an outpouring of books and journal articles concerned with the elusive concept of cultural competence and how it could be developed in practitioners.

In the UK clinical professionals, particularly in disciplines such as psychiatry and midwifery, were becoming concerned about their ability to provide appropriate and effective care for the growing numbers of ethnic minority clients that were presenting, particularly to secondary care institutions (Rack 1982). Some of these clinical professionals expressed views forthrightly (*pace* gender diversity!).

> For the practitioner the question of whether the minorities ought, or ought not, to remain ethnically different should be irrelevant. The fact is that they are. Insofar as his specialism, whatever it is, demands that he should take into account the social and cultural worlds in which his clients live, he needs to make a response to ethnic diversity. If he does not, his practice is inadequate in purely professional terms. (Ballard 1979)

Yet it was not until the late 1980s and early 1990s that there was the beginning of research and some publication in the UK about issues of race and health and the connections with culture and competence. In *Nursing in a multi-ethnic society: a selected annotated bibliography*, Gerrish et al (1996) make two very important points.

> An attempt has been made to identify empirical research in the field of nursing and midwifery practice and education, however there appears to be comparatively little published and much of what has been published is of a small scale. This raises questions regarding the generalisability of findings to different settings, particularly when considering the relevance of North American literature to the British context.

The cultural competence model

and later:

The paucity of British literature in comparison to that from North America most probably reflects the relatively recent concern with these issues in the UK.

It is salutary to reflect on the gap between Ballard's and Rack's concerns in the 1970s, Baxter's warnings in the 1980s of the likely consequences of the hardships faced by black and ethnic minority nurses and the recent findings of Beishon et al (1995) and Gerrish et al (1996) and the fact that there has been so little interest and research in the area of cultural competence in the UK.

Gerrish et al (1996) followed up their annotated bibliography with *Nursing in a multi-ethnic society*, in which they outlined the results of a 2-year study commissioned by the ENB on the education and preparation of nurses and midwives for work in the UK. In this, they point to the fact that although the law governing the content of nursing and midwifery education, passed in 1979, had been amended in 1989 to include a requirement that all nurses demonstrate 'an appreciation of the influence of social, political and *cultural* factors in relation to health care', neither the ENB nor the UKCC, provided very much specific guidance on how this was to be achieved or to what level or standard.

CRITICAL VIEWS

In the USA there have been critics of the melting pot theory of social evolution and its influence on the development of a culturally competent model of care. Glynn & Rockarts (1986) challenge the approval of this model of societal development and point out that it is predicated on an assimilationist view of various ethnic groups and their ultimate subsumption into the concept of being American. Along with others, they were influential in the acceptance of the fact that there was not a democratic 'one size fits all' style of American nursing delivered equitably to all Americans, whatever their ethnic or cultural inheritance. They also further raised concern about cultural competence and particularly its inclusion in nursing curricula:

> Only as such concepts are cognitively and affectively understood and integrated clinically by everyone involved will the multicultural dimension of nursing care become a viable reality and not just an academic exercise.

Lynam (1992) expresses concern that the emphasis on competence in nursing curricula could lead to too much n being included which could encourage nurses to stere patients based on their training and therefore cause them to ig the other variables such as class, age, gender and intercultural v ations which might cause this particular patient to be differe. Gerrish et al (1996) are at pains to point out that it is not enough fo. the practitioner to seek to become more skilled in transcultural communication and care but that the NHS itself must examine its institutional involvement in delivery of inappropriate health care and in the continuation of discriminatory practices.

ROLES

There are many 'players' in the development of cultural competence as a viable concept, particularly in the UK. These include:

- the government of the day
- the executive of the NHS
- the professional bodies
- educational institutions
- the practitioner
- the client/user/patient.

The government of the day

Over the last 20 years there have been many policy statements aimed at improving the health care experience of and outcomes for ethnic minority clients. In each of the major White Papers of recent times, there has been a major section or emphasis on the need to deal with the 'problem' of ethnic minority health or health care services.

The executive of the NHS

In interpreting and implementing Department of Health policy, the NHS Executive or the NHS Management Executive has relied on time- and cash-limited initiatives (as it does for all its implementations), such as:

- the NHS Ethnic Health Unit
- the Women's Unit
- the Equal Opportunity Unit.

All of these bodies have lobbied for, provided or funded educational and research projects and tried to ensure that ethnic minority individuals fare better in their interactions with the NHS, whether as staff or clients.

The professional bodies

Both the ENB and the UKCC as well as unions such as UNISON have espoused policies that seek to improve the health care experience for ethnic minority workers and patients. The UKCC was the commissioner of the work by Gerrish et al (1996) which looked initially at the literature and research current available in the USA and the UK and, over 2 years, investigated the preparation that nurses were given to enable them to function in a multiethnic society.

Educational institutions

The educational establishment responsible for providing training for nurses is now usually firmly part of a university faculty. This came about after the implementation of Project 2000 which radically shifted the education of nurses away from 'on-the-job' training to a much more theoretical initial base. Because of the requirement that all colleges of further education become attached to universities, these former Colleges of Health are now no longer attached to the local health authority but to the university. However, the ENB's own research publication is at pains to point out, in its assessments of curricula under this new regime, that 'Curriculum documents express ambitious programme aims. ... Some programmes are more appropriately organised than others to achieve these aims' (ENB 1996).

There is very little evidence of structured work to improve the cultural competence of nurses being developed for the future and compliance with the letter of the law allows institutions to provide training to suit their local community, which can mean that students trained for a national service in one part of the country may have little or no knowledge of ethnic minorities, particularly because of the common tendency to undercount in areas where there are few ethnic minority individuals (Cooper 1996).

The other tack taken by the educational institutions is based on getting a higher number of students from ethnic minority communities into nursing. Bharj (1995) in particular looks at the reasons why so few Asian people see nursing as a viable or desirable career option.

The practitioner

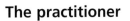

In most of the literature on cultural competence, the onus appears to have been equally placed upon the practitioner and the educational institutions to deal with the problems of ethnic minority health. All writers, whether practitioner, researcher or educator, are explicit about the responsibility of the practitioner to change and they offer various models of the ideally culturally competent practitioner (Campinha-Bacote 1994a, b, Gerrish et al 1996, Kim 1992). There are also high expectations that ethnic minority practitioners, by their presence, will automatically make a difference to the cultural competence of the organisation within which they are located (Manzoor 1995).

The client/user/patient

The receiver of health care, particularly in the USA, is no longer expected to become a proto-American but is able to be an individual citizen with behavioural, cultural, social and genetic inheritances and differences that are as valid as anyone else's (Glynn & Rockarts 1986). In the UK there is the dissonance of the pledge to treat each person equally and the cultural imposition inherent in this approach. There has also always been a reluctance in Britain to allow separate provision, be it of schools or of health care, because this is easily pointed out as preferential treatment and liable to damage the electoral chances of any candidate, local or national, who was seen to support it. However, as the 'ethnic vote' became more and more important, particularly in inner cities or marginal seats, more and more funding for voluntary organisations became available. These organisations, particularly in mental health provision, enabled the development and explicit specification of the services required by ethnic minority clients. It is often these voluntary organisations which have served as working models for the individual client to specify what he or she means by cultural competence (Rack 1982).

STAGES

The societal, organisational and personal stages of cultural competence seem to mirror each other. The lag or overlap from societal to organisational to personal depends upon the national culture in which the organisation in question is based (Hofstede 1980). In the

The cultural competence model

USA the trend has been from the melting pot assimilationist view to the present one of respect for individual cultural differences (Glynn & Rockarts 1986). In the UK, while there has never been an espousal of the melting pot theory, there was at best a focus on equality for all which required acculturation by the ethnic minorities but not acceptance by the ethnic majority (Gerrish et al 1996). While Tate (1996) points to the long list of studies over the last 30 years and the similarity of response to each ('… *a flurry of defensive activity which subsides as the reports become old news*'), there is certainly a determination to keep the issue at the forefront of educational and practice agendas by Tate herself and other commentators such as Bharj, Gerrish, Husband, Mackenzie and Manzoor.

The stage at which cultural competence appears to be in the UK at present is one of political acceptance of the validity of the concept but a lack of practical implementation initiatives or true benefit realisation frameworks. Organisations are exhorted to become culturally competent with no guidance as to how this could be done, except that employing more ethnic minority staff is the way forward. In the meantime, cultural competence as a useful concept is becoming in danger of acquiring the business jargon status of '*the learning organisation*', or '*the information culture*'.

ASSESSMENT

There have been few studies of cultural competence of nurses in the USA. Griepp (1996) reports on a study of ethnocentrism based on a study of 268 practising nurses which found that there was ingroup favouritism and that it was difficult to assess the effect of covert bias in this type of study. The author recommends direct observation studies as the ideal way of objective study but points out their prohibitive expense. A study of knowledge and attitudes of nurses towards ethnic minority clients by Rooda (1993) used a final survey sample of 274 white nurses. While the community had 37% ethnic minorities, the researchers excluded the 11% of their sample that was from ethnic minority respondents but retained the 'small number' of males. The findings, unsurprisingly, showed nurses of one ethnic group are more likely to be biased towards clients from that ethnic group. Even the author admits the flaws in this study.

There have been no studies in the UK which have looked at the level of cultural competence among nurses. Studies such as

Beishon et al (1995) have shown that the organisation in which most ethnic minority nurses work, the NHS, has serious problems in the gap between written policies on employment and equal opportunity, and the actual practice. Gerrish et al's (1996) study is based on an assessment of the difference between policy and practice of the inclusion of culturally specific modules in nurse training by 55 institutions.

EVALUATION

There is nothing in the literature, either in the USA or in the UK, that provides an evaluation of cultural competence. It is a point well made by Gerrish et al (1994) that there is no empirical research in this area in the UK.

DESIGNS AND MODELS

Stubbs (1993) proposes a multiculturalist, ethnic sensitivity model in which greater knowledge of different cultures, with improved skills in crosscultural communication and with the creation of particular ethnic specialisms, leads to service improvement.

The model proposed by Culley (1996) states that it is essential for nurses and nurse educators to assist practitioners to identify ways in which they can listen to and work with minority ethnic communities. Nurses and nurse educators need to contextualise the health of minority ethnic groups, exploring the dynamics of discriminatory practices which structure many aspects of everyday life. She concludes that health professionals would be greatly aided in this task by research which focused on complex ways in which race, culture, gender, age and socioeconomic dimensions may interact in influencing both patterns of health status and utilisation of health services.

The conceptual model of cultural competence in psychiatric nursing, first described by Campinha-Bacote in 1994, states that cultural competence is a process which contains four logical work areas for the individual, the organization and society (Fig. 9.1).

Where the 'cultural competence' model proposed by Campinha-Bacote differs from its predecessors is in its absolute conviction that what is being proposed is a process and that this process begins and ends with the individual, taking in the organisation, the nation and the world on its way. In this conceptual

The cultural competence model

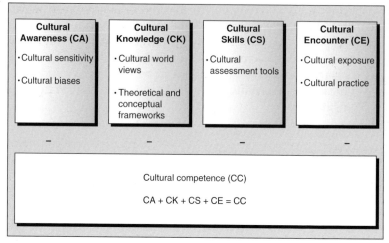

Figure 9.1 Conceptual model of cultural competence (after Campinha-Bacote 1994a).

model of cultural competence, the psychiatric nurse '... sees herself or himself always in the process of *becoming* culturally competent rather than *being* culturally competent' (Campinha-Bacote 1994a). This process does not strive for the finished perfection of some other models but is seen rather as a personal process, as much guided by the practitioner as by teachers and role models.

Thus while cultural awareness involves becoming more aware and open to other cultures, it is not in the quaint or 'National Geographic' style but in terms of gauging one's own tendency to 'cultural imposition' (Leininger 1978) or in terms of understanding one's own interpersonal style. Leininger described cultural imposition as the tendency to assume that the ethnic majority view, standards and beliefs are naturally superior and the norm. All else is deviance and the problem of the 'deviant' group.

Campinha-Bacote also uses Bell & Evans' (1981) descriptions of five interpersonal styles to further explain her model.

- *Overt hostility* – interactions are played out against a background of hostility and hatred and often with a power imbalance in favour of the practitioner.
- *Covert prejudice* – where the hostility and hatred are just as deep seated but fear of the consequences of revealing them makes any expression hidden and even harder to challenge.
- *Cultural ignorance* – the nurse knows so little about a particular client's cultural group that he or she is immobilised by fear of ineptitude or xenophobia.

- *Colour blind* – the 'we treat everybody the same' school of multiethnic practice. This of course leads into the trap of cultural imposition and makes any complaint or non-compliance from an ethnic minority client seem like ungrateful whingeing or special pleading.
- *Culturally liberated* – this does not mean that nurses are the perfect multiethnic practitioners but that they are aware of their responses to different ethnic groups and cultural manifestations and guard against these having a negative impact upon the care relationship.

Bell & Evans also describe four different types of interacting styles within any cultural group.

- *Acculturated* – the individual consciously rejects their cultural inheritance and identifies almost totally with the majority cultural view.
- *Culturally immersed* – the individual totally rejects the majority cultural view and clings to their cultural inheritance.
- *Traditional interacting* – neither accepting or rejecting their own or the majority culture. However, will not reveal beliefs easily.
- *Bicultural interacting* – this individual values and understands their own cultural inheritance and feels comfortable with it but is also able to see that this might be so for others and actively enjoys living and working in a diverse community.

The conceptual model of 'cultural communicative competence' discussed by Gerrish et al (1996) is a practical synthesis of the concepts of 'cultural communicative competence' and 'intercultural communicative competence' developed in the work of Kim (1992). It is proposed that the knowledge base built up by the individual practitioner about other cultures is added to grounding in the differences between cultures and modes of communication.

IMPLEMENTATION OF CULTURAL COMPETENCE TRAINING PROGRAMMES

Although there is a requirement, as stated before, that nursing training programmes should include training that would fit the qualified nurse to serve the local community, we have seen that this is a policy more planned for than implemented and Gerrish et al (1996) found:

> Overall the questionnaire survey of curricula content has generated a sense that many programmes have begun to address the issue of

The cultural competence model

how to prepare members of the nursing professions to work in a multi-ethnic society. However, the data leave no room for complacency. A number of institutions felt able to declare that there was no ethnic minority community in their locality; hence it was not an issue for them. Other responses strongly suggested that a barely tokenistic acknowledgement of the challenge of ethnic diversity had been put in place.

This literature survey has been unable to identify any published research on the question of programmes of training for practitioners already qualified and working in the NHS.

BELIEFS AND ASSUMPTIONS IN CULTURAL COMPETENCE

The three key beliefs and assumptions that are pertinent here are as follows.

First, that there is such an entity or skill as cultural competence and that its acquisition is possible with greater or lesser degrees of effort (Campinha-Bacote 1994, Gerrish et al 1996, Leininger 1978, Rack 1982).

Second, that it is possible and desirable to provide training to improve the cultural competence of nurses and that this will in turn improve the cultural competence of the health care organisations in which these nurses eventually work (Bharj 1995, ENB 1993, Gerrish et al 1996, Glynn & Rackarts 1986, Rooda 1993, Thorpe & Baker 1995).

And third, that the employment of higher numbers of ethnic minority health care staff, particularly nurses, will improve the overall cultural competence of the NHS (Bharj 1995, Gerrish et al 1996, Manzoor 1995, 1996, Tate 1996).

KEY COMPONENTS OF CULTURAL COMPETENCE

The key components of all the models or concepts of cultural competence discussed can be summed up as follows.

- Acceptance of difference as normal, and only to be expected, for human beings.
- Acceptance of the inherent right of all residents in a society to identify as part of the society and acceptance of the resultant changes.

- The acquisition of knowledge about other cultures.
- A learning stance.

References

Ballard C 1979 Conflict, continuity and change: second generation South Asians. In: Khan S (ed) Minority families in Britain: support and stress. Macmillan, London

Beckhard R, Harris R T 1987 Organisational transitions. Addison-Wesley, Reading, MA

Beishon S, Virdee S, Hagell A 1995 Nursing in a multi-ethnic NHS. Policy Studies Institute, London

Bell, Evans 1981 Cited in Campinha-Bacote 1994a

Bharj K K 1995 Nurse recruitment: an Asian response. University of Bradford, Bradford

Bower M 1966 The will to manage. McGraw-Hill, New York

Campinha-Bacote J 1994a Cultural competence in psychiatric mental health nursing: a conceptual model. Nursing Clinics of North America 29(1):1–8

Campinha-Bacote J 1994b Transcultural psychiatric nursing: diagnostic and treatment issues. Journal of Psychosocial Nursing 32(8):41–46

Cooper C 1996 Rural racism under attack. Community Care (113); 28th March–3rd April, pp 9–10

Culley L 1996 A critique of multiculturalism in healthcare: the challenge for nurse education. Journal of Advanced Nursing 23:564–570

Devore W, Schlesinger F G 1981 Ethnic-sensitive social work practice. C V Mosby, St Louis

English National Board 1996 The evaluation of pre-registration undergraduate degrees in nursing and midwifery. ENB, London

Gerrish K, Husband C, Mackenzie J 1996 Nursing in a multi-ethnic society. Open University Press, Buckingham

Glynn N J, Rockarts B G 1986 Multiculturalism in nursing: implications for faculty development. Journal of Nursing Education 25(1):39–41

Griepp M 1996 Culture, age and gender: effects on quality of a predicated self and colleague reactions. International Journal of Nursing Studies 33(1):83–97

Hofstede G 1980 Culture's consequences. In: Pugh D S, Hickson D J (eds) Writers on organizations. Penguin, London

Kim Y Y 1992 Intercultural communication competence: a systems theoretic view. In: Gudykunst W B, Kim Y Y (eds) Readings on communications with strangers. McGraw-Hill, New York

Leininger M 1967 The culture concept and its relevance to nursing. Journal of Nursing Education 6(2):27

Leininger M 1978 Transcultural nursing: concepts, theories and practices. Wiley, New York

Lum D 1986 Social work practice and people of color. Brooks/Cole, California

Lynam J 1992 Towards the goal of providing culturally sensitive care: principles upon which to build nursing curricula. Journal of Advanced Nursing 17:149–157

The cultural competence model

Manzoor Z 1995 Nurse recruitment: an Asian response. University of Bradford, Bradford

Manzoor Z 1996 From policy to practice. Nursing Standard 10(28):8

Miller S 1993 In: Harrison R (ed) Human resource management: issues and strategies. Addison-Wesley, London

Minzberg H 1983 Power in and around organisations. Prentice Hall, New York

Ouchi W 1981 Theory Z: how American business can meet the Japanese challenge. Addison-Wesley, New York

Rack P 1982 Race, culture and mental disorder. Routledge, London

Rooda L A 1993 Knowledge and attitudes of nurses toward culturally different patients: implications for nursing education. Journal of Nursing Education 32(5):209–213

Stubbs P 1993 'Ethnically sensitive' or 'anti-racist'? Models for health research and service delivery. In: Ahmad W I U (ed) Race and health in contemporary Britain. Open University Press, Buckingham

Tate C W 1996 Equal opportunities. Race into action. Nursing Times 92(22): 28–30

Thorpe D E, Baker C P 1995 Addressing 'cultural competence' in healthcare education. Paediatric Physical Therapy 143–144

Wells S A 1995 Creating a culturally competent workforce. Caring Magazine 50–53

Young C A 1997 District nurse competencies: a Bradford perspective. MA dissertation, Nuffield Institute

Further reading

Amos V 1996 An uphill task. Nursing Standard 10(29):19

Begum N 1995 Beyond samosas and reggae: a guide to developing services for black disabled people. King's Fund, London

Begum N 1995 Improving disability services: the way forward for health and social services. King's Fund, London

Crowley J J, Simmons S 1992 Mental health, race and ethnicity: a retrospective study of the care of ethnic minorities and whites in a psychiatric unit. Journal of Advanced Nursing 17:1078–1087

Department of Health 1996 Responding to diversity: a study of commissioning issues and good practice in purchasing minority ethnic health. Office for Public Health Management, London

Easton L 1996 Inquiry as black staff leave hospital jobs. Nursing Times 22(21):6

Eleftheriadou Z 1966 In: Lloyd M, Bor R (eds) Communication with patients from different cultural backgrounds. Churchill Livingstone, Edinburgh, pp 85–103

Fatchett A 1996 Turning fiction into fact. Nursing Standard 10(29):24–25

Fernando S 1995 Mental health in a multi-ethnic society: a multidisciplinary handbook. Routledge, London

Foster P 1996 Inequalities in health: what health systems can and cannot do. Journal of Health Services Research and Policy 1(3):179–182

Fry A J, Nguyen T 1996 Culture and the self: implications for the perception of depression by Australian and Vietnamese nursing students. Journal of Advanced Nursing 23:1147–1154

Healy P 1996 Equality matters. Nursing Standard 10(29):22–23

Healy P 1996 Ethnic purchasing advice is a success. Nursing Standard 10(22):9

Jarrold K 1996 Ethnic minority staff in the NHS – a programme of action. EL 96(4). NHSE, London

King M B 1991 Transcultural psychiatry. Medicine International 95:3978–3980

Kumar A 1996 In: Matthew L (ed) Cultural issues in the care of mentally ill Asian elders. Chapman and Hall, London, pp 182–204

Leifer D 1996 Ethnic minorities get restricted priorities. Nursing Standard 10(34):8

Leisten R, Richardson J 1996 The ethnicity question. Journal of Community Nursing 10(4):28–29

McKenzie K, Crowcroft N 1996 Ethnicity, race, and culture: guidelines for research, audit and publication. British Medical Journal 312:1094

NHS Centre for Reviews and Dissemination 1996 Ethnicity and health: reviews of literature and guidance for purchasers in the areas of cardiovascular disease mental health, and haemoglobinopathies. University of York, York

Pringle M, Rothera I 1996 Practicality of recording patient ethnicity in general practice: descriptive intervention study and attitude survey. British Medical Journal 312:1080–1082

Tullmann D F 1992 Cultural diversity in nursing education: does it affect racism in the nursing profession? Journal of Nursing Education 31(7)

The cultural competence model

Application **9:1**

Sonia Harding

Reviewing and redesigning a Trust's equal opportunities policy: a personal account from Newham Community Health Services

INTRODUCTION

Newham Community Health Services NHS Trust operates in one of the poorest London boroughs, with a highly diverse population, so it faces a greater range of challenges than most. I have worked in the health services in this district for the past 18 years, as a general nurse, midwife and health visitor. Since becoming a trust in 1995, the organisation has had a programme for developing equal opportunities and has won a Department of Health Equalities award for its work on health and race. In 1999, it also won the *Health Service Journal* Trust of the Year Award.

My last post as a locality service manager was instrumental in extending my thinking from a standpoint which addressed itself primarily to the needs of the individual to one which more readily embraced a population's perspective. This wider approach brought with it a heightened awareness and concern for the wider issues of fairness and equal opportunities. After several years in my role as a team manager I got to the stage where I was ready for a new challenge and developing my emerging interest in equal opportunities seemed to be one direction I could take. I replied to the trust advertisement for candidates for the Black and Ethnic Minority Leadership (BEL) Development Programme. This was a 1-year programme run by the King's Fund which offered personal, organisational and mentor development experience for black and ethnic minority staff, including nurses G grade and above who were looking to go into their first management post. In late 1997 I became one of three Newham participants to the programme. Taking a closer look at what was on offer in the programme, the personal and mentor developmental aspects particularly appealed to me. The organisational development strand, however, presented me with the opportunity to realise a professional interest in equal opportunities.

My joining the BEL programme coincided with an organisational development audit within my trust. As part of the BEL Programme my project was identified from this work in agreement with the Chair of the Health and Race Task Group and the Director of Human Resources. This would be to 'review and redesign the trust's equal opportunities policy, taking account of the existing mechanism for dealing with breaches of the policy and the absence of racial, sexual and other harassment policies'.

Grappling with the complex and sensitive nature of this area of work has been greatly rewarding and I would like to share some of the challenges and outcomes and my learning from this.

FINDING A FRAMEWORK

Confronted with the question of where to start and what models to apply to my approach, one of the first publications I came across was *Racial equality means business: a standard for racial equality for employers*. The standard comprised a checklist which summarises the range of actions an organisation needs to consider when planning and implementing a racial equality programme. It had been produced some 2 years earlier (1995) by the Commission for Racial Equality but was still highly relevant and became the framework for the approach I was to use in developing my work.

The standard helps organisations to:

- assess their current position and commitment to the development of equality strategies
- consider the range of organisational actions needed to achieve change
- understand the outcomes which must be achieved and demonstrated.

The use of this guide enabled me to consider objectively the intentions of the review which were to:

- discover the views of staff, the trust board and external partners on the present policy
- explore whether a new policy was needed

Managing change: diversity, the key to success

Box 9.1.1 Questionnaire used in interviews

- Are staff given the opportunity to develop and take risk?*
- How is equality of opportunity and the management of diversity being implemented in your organisation and how are you involved?*
- Do you know if the trust has an equal opportunity policy? Have you seen it? Have you read it?
- How have you implemented the policy in your service area?
- Do you think there is a clear commitment at the highest level of the trust in emphasising the value placed on equality of opportunity?
- How can this policy be improved?
- What do you think are the priority areas for change and improvement?
- What do you consider should be the aims and objectives of the organisation in terms of equality of opportunity?
- Can you suggest ways in which the policy can be implemented?
- What types of positive action programmes can be introduced to Newham to the benefit of staff and the community?
- How can the trust ensure equal opportunity issues are taken account of in matters of finance and contracting?
- What is your role in the monitoring of this policy?
- What strategies do you have in place for ensuring everyone owns the policy?
- What issues does your policy address specifically and why?*
- What do you consider should be the aims and objectives of the policy?*
- What do you see as the cost of not having an EO policy?*

*Additional questions asked of external organisations

- gain an understanding of what the structure/framework of a new policy for the trust could be
- gain an understanding of how a new policy should be promoted in the trust.

Using a semi-structured questionnaire (see Box 9.1.1) I interviewed 40 staff from within the trust and seven public and private managers in a number of other organisations. The internal interviews were with a cross-section of managers and staff from a range of services and included a trade union representative, health visitors, school nurses, support services, senior clinical managers and general managers together with non-executive and executive members of the trust board. Interviews sought information about their knowledge and understanding and opinions about equal opportunities policies and development within the trust. The purpose of interviewing people outside the trust was to elicit managers' views on developing commitment to equality of opportunity and the barriers they had encountered in managing a diverse workforce, particularly in developing ownership of policies and procedures which tackle inequalities. External interviewees in the public sector consisted of the Director of the NHS Executive's Equal Opportunities Unit programme Positively Diverse (see Application 10.1, p 247), human resource managers from the local health authority and social services department and a nurse with responsibility for equal opportunities within a primary care group. Private sector organisations were represented by human resource managers from the Midland Bank and Ford Motor Company.

VIEWS FROM THE EXTERNAL ORGANISATIONS

Managers in the public and private organisations outside the trust emphasised the need for policies which had a clear strategy and a common purpose and were consistent in application to all employees within the trust. It was also suggested that policies should provide sound guidance with regard to individual responsibilities and obligations to each other, this being seen as fundamental to developing staff commitment. Managers also felt it was vital to learn from and to celebrate differences in the organisation.

VIEWS FROM TRUST STAFF

The trust staff expected a policy which supported them in taking positive actions in their dealings with their colleagues and clients. It was important to them that the policy:

- clearly stated the support available to deal with any breach of equality of opportunity
- clearly outlined responsibilities for the management of the policy
- clearly stated clients' responsibilities
- outlined how staff will be supported in dealing with abuse from clients
- was written in a user-friendly manner
- highlighted the need for training for all on issues of equality of opportunity
- outlined clear lines of communication as part of a strategy to disseminate the policy to service users and visitors.

VIEWS FROM TRUST MANAGERS

Managers within the trust expected to have a policy which supported them and the staff in finding a way through the issues and concerns around equal opportunities. They expected to have a policy which:

The Newham approach and policies

- outlined the values of the trust
- would cover the full range of disadvantaged groups
- reflected the organisation's relationship with the wider community
- was clearly written and easy to understand
- had clear lines of accountability
- would take account of the needs of both staff and managers.

During the course of this work, the trust accepted an invitation from the NHS Equal Opportunities Unit to be one of the 40 national reference sites for the Positively Diverse programme. This programme had the principal aim of mainstreaming equal opportunities within the NHS by developing the capacity of managers with designated responsibility for this area of activity to manage change. It seemed appropriate for me to apply for the post. However, this took some soul searching. I had up to this point taken very few risks in my working life. I thought about uncertainties in terms of the lack of job security, the move to a new area of work, the overall dilemmas and pitfalls which seemed to be a feature of work in equalities. However, the knowledge, skills and network I had gained from my involvement in the BEL project helped me to appreciate development opportunities which could be an outcome of this work. I thus felt confident that the risks associated with this change of employment were outweighed by the benefits.

OUTPUTS AND OUTCOMES

Over the 2-year period we developed two policy documents: an Equal Opportunity Policy and Guidelines on Valuing Diversity and Ensuring Dignity in the Workplace. We also developed an action plan which was based on the results of the Positively Diverse audit. These documents reflected and emphasised the trust's human resource strategy that the employees and the community of Newham matter and have the right to be:

- shown respect, appreciation and consideration
- given a fair hearing at all times
- dealt with courteously, with civility and politeness
- given honest feedback.

The policies provide clear statements of the:

- trust's commitment to the eradication of harassment and discrimination
- positive behaviours expected of each individual in the organisation
- individual and group responsibilities in achieving the aims of the policy
- provision of staff support

- management and investigation of breaches
- monitoring and reporting arrangements to measure progress.

The policies were agreed by the trust board and the Joint Staff Consultative Committee and launched in November 1999. At the launch of the policies we had a 'question time' event with national and local figures who are committed to issues of equal opportunity and the management and valuing of diversity. This signalled to staff the commitment of the trust to this strategy. On the same day the trust became winners of the title of Trust of the Year in the *Health Service Journal*'s 18th Annual Health Management Awards. We were highly rated by the judges for the development of some imaginative partnerships and collaborative relationships and were cited as standing out in leadership and management. We were judged as generating a distinctive organisational ethos which was felt to be laudable in the context of our socioeconomically deprived environment.

CONCLUSION

Our policies are employee centred and, together with the action plan on diversity, are the start of translating our aspiration to be a 'good equal opportunities employer' into action. Although policies will not of themselves prevent unfair, unequal and disadvantageous treatment, they will support individual employees and the organisation in solving the difficulties encountered in providing services which the community wants and will use. We will know how effective these policies are in meeting both staff and managers' needs through the reviews and monitoring we will be undertaking.

We are acutely aware that the process is not complete. One year on, however, there is a distinct feeling that equality of opportunity is now within everyone's consciousness. The open debate, although sometimes painful, is happening and is all part of the complexity of managing and valuing diversity.

At a personal level, I have experienced tremendous benefits, not least the acquisition of a wide range of new skills, particularly in carrying out the audit and in presenting the information to staff in an effective way. I am better able to shoulder high levels of responsibility and am reassured that individuals can make a difference in a complex organisation. I have gained confidence in my ability to be involved in the process of change and have taken the challenges as an invitation to try and not to be silent.

The Newham approach and policies

Application **9:2**

Barbara Burford

A framework for change: the case of the Charter NHS Trust

TRUST PROFILE

This NHS trust provides acute, community and mental health services. It was created 2 years ago from the merger of two existing trusts, giving a workforce of 5000. The trust comprises urban and rural communities and is generally affluent but with pockets of deprivation. There is also a significant proportion of minority ethnic groups within the community. The merger created a single organisation from different cultures and involved merging policies and procedures, appointing staff to senior positions, loss of staff through voluntary redundancy, early retirement and natural turnover. Communication throughout the trust was a priority during restructuring and staff generally felt well informed about changes.

There is a shortage of nursing staff: the trust's recent European recruitment drive has boosted joiners but recruitment in general does not match the level of leavers. Exit interviews have shown a variety of reasons for leaving but many noted low morale and lack of team working. Winter pressures and a flu epidemic have added to the pressures on all staff and communication has suffered as a result.

Charter considered itself an equal opportunities employer and that it 'saw its staff as its most valued resource'. Within a year it had signed up to become a national reference site for a Department of Health organisational development programme which works with trusts to ensure mainstreaming of equality of opportunity and diversity into their core service functionality. As part of its strategy in managing diversity, the trust undertook an audit of the whole workforce.

AUDIT RESULTS

The trust was surprised and disappointed at what it found. Whilst junior professional and administrative posts tend to mirror the ethnic distribution in the population this is not reflected in senior professional or managerial positions (Table 9.2.1). Another finding of the audit was hidden disability within the workforce (Table 9.2.2). Further audit results are as follows.

- Junior grades reflect the community profile; senior grades do not.
- Awareness of policies on redundancy and transfer or redeployment is relatively low (60% and 40% respectively).
- Awareness of policies on health and safety, disciplinary matters and grievances is high (95%, 90% and 90% respectively).

Table 9.2.1 Percentage of ethnic groups in workforce and in community

Ethnic group	% in community	% in workforce
White	79	76
Black – Caribbean	8	10
Black – African	3	4
Black – other	1	1
Asian	7	8
Other	2	1

Table 9.2.2 Percentage of persons with disability in workforce and in community

Disability status	% in community	% in workforce
1. Registered disabled		1
2. Disabled but not registered		1
3. Having a disability requiring support in the workplace		2
4. Having a disability which occasionally affects your work		4
Total	9*	8

*Estimate but not directly comparable with workforce figures. Community disability figures are likely to underestimate categories 3 and 4.

A framework for change

● 45% of white staff think there is a clear public commitment at the highest level of their organisation to equal opportunities; 30% of minority ethnic staff share this view.

● 60% of white staff feel that commitment to equal opportunity is clear to employees; 40% of minority ethnic staff agree.

● 40% of white staff and 35% of minority ethnic employees think the commitment to equal opportunities is made clear to patients.

● 30% of staff from ethnic minority groups say they have been harassed or bullied on grounds of race in the last 12 months.

● 15% of all staff say they have been harassed or bullied on grounds of gender and 5% on grounds of age.

● Of staff who say they have some disability, 15% say they have experienced harassment or bullying because of it in the last 12 months.

● Supervisors or managers are cited as the main sources of gender harassment (25%) and of harassment due to disability (40%). Other team members and patients/clients are also major sources.

● The main source of racial harassment for minority ethnic staff is also attributed to supervisors or managers (25%).

● 60% of all respondents do not think staff feel appreciated: this does not vary significantly for different ethnic groups, gender or disability.

● 28% of white staff and 22% of minority ethnic respondents feel staff are confident about expressing their views and concerns.

TAKING ACTION FOR CHANGE

Following the audit the trust felt it necessary to question and address:

● what was really meant by 'an equal opportunities employer' and 'our staff are our most valued resource' (these were stated as underpinning values in its equal opportunities policy)

● whether the equal opportunities aspirations of the Executive were reflected in action throughout the organisation

● what the trust should do about it.

In an organisation such as the NHS which is people intensive and knowledge driven, any action or development which has an effect upon its key resource, its staff, must be informed, linked with and ultimately driven by the key strategic drivers of the entire organisation. Key strategic issues for the trust include the implementation of the following.

● *Clinical governance* – a mechanism to facilitate the accounting for and improve the quality and the standard of patient care.

Managing change: diversity, the key to success

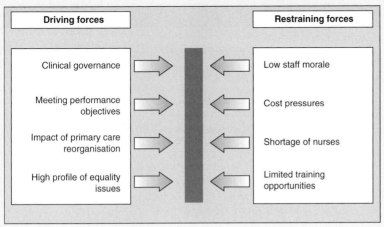

Figure 9.2.1   Main local forces

- *National Service Frameworks* – establishing a clearer evidence base for services and the benchmarking of performances.
- *The reorganisation of primary care* – the new management structures within primary care teams and the requirement for increased collaboration between sectors.
- *Working Together* – the government's national agenda for local implementation to develop the human resource capability within the NHS.
- *The Vital Connection*, the NHS Equal Opportunities Framework – setting out the standards, targets, guidance and support available for the service in ensuring equality for staff and thereby improving equity in service delivery.

In achieving these objectives the main local forces are those shown in Figure 9.2.1.

Specific areas which the trust felt it had to address as priorities are as follows.

- Confidence to express concerns is low. How can the trust ensure that contentious issues are discussed and resolved within the organisation and not in the media or courts?
- What actions might the trust take to increase the numbers from ethnic minority groups in senior positions?
- How is the trust's disability profile significant in providing quality clinical care to all sections of the community?

To achieve this, actions so far have included those shown in Box 9.2.1.

Box 9.2.1

General

● Human resource policies have been reviewed and consolidated across the organisation, in consultation with staff and their representatives.

● Associated with this, managers have been asked to familiarise themselves with all policies.

● Equal opportunities has been addressed in all induction training and management programmes.

Ethnic minorities

● A Job Shop in the community run by staff who might be considered role models for minority ethnic groups has boosted applicants from ethnic minority groups.

Disability

● Physical access has been reviewed, principally for patients and wheelchair access provided to all patient areas.

● Induction loops have been fitted to wards for elderly patients, in the boardroom and all training rooms.

DISCUSSION

Many trusts can identify with Charter. It has good management, it has been through the merger, joined up to go through organisational development and taken actions to address priorities. It is not perfect and communications suffer when under pressure. It is committed to equal opportunities but not yet achieving its ambitions on harassment and bullying and low levels of staff from ethnic minorities in senior positions.

The strategic issues and pressures are those of providing quality health care. This aims to encourage the view that a diverse workforce 'fit for purpose' must be seen as central for achieving these core strategic business and organisational objectives rather than as something to think about when time and resources allow. On general actions taken by the trust, managers have been asked to familiarise themselves with all policies. This is intentionally weak and may raise the issue of ongoing training for managers.

Points to think about include:

● conformance with legal obligations
● the role and social responsibility of the NHS as an employer
● releasing the potential of the workforce
● the cost of poor retention and lack of development
● costs and savings of proposed actions
● who owns equal opportunities?

- who leads it?
- where does it sit within the organisation?

The relatively low levels of ethnic minority staff could be related back to levels of harassment and lack of confidence in expressing concerns and the effect that these factors may have on the progression of staff to more senior positions. Where are the role models?

When addressing disability, an important consideration should be the cost of early retirement versus making it possible to continue work. The proportion of employees with a disability is similar to the proportion in the community. Has the trust met its commitment to equal opportunities in this area?

KEY LEARNING AND ACTION POINTS

General management issues

Learning points

- It is important to build on a good baseline audit which will highlight areas for further investigation.
- More information and better understanding are crucial in all areas but this should not be used as an excuse for not doing anything.
- Providing support and training for managers is crucial, otherwise identified improvements will not happen.

Action points

- Any progress needs clear commitment from the top.
- The Board needs to be seen to lead from the front: encouraging discussion, visible at diversity workshops, establishing a programme of change, promoting action groups.

Ensuring that contentious issues are discussed and resolved within the organisation and not in the media or courts

Learning points

- There is a need to balance long-term organisational (cultural) change with the needs of individuals and problems encountered by those dealing with critical incidents.
- Actions need to be followed through if credibility is to be maintained.

A framework for change

Action points

- Find out where the real problems lie: circumstances are likely to vary, requiring a variety of solutions to address them.
- Managers require new HR capabilities before the confidence of individuals they manage can be expected to rise. Development of standards and training of managers are required.
- There are various mechanisms for empowering staff: workshops, flyers, assertiveness skills, staff charter, involvement policy, expression of concern procedure, guarantees of confidentiality.

External facilitators, for example the Advisory, Conciliatory and Arbitration Service (ACAS), Citizens Advice Bureau, trade unions and staff counselling have a role.

Increasing the numbers from ethnic minority groups in senior positions

Learning points

- It is within the organisation's gift to break through a glass ceiling: hidden bias within working practices as well as selection and promotion procedures need to be challenged.
- The results of the audit can be used to challenge assumptions and promote action.
- It is essential to share findings openly and widely throughout the trust, supported by a board-level action plan.

Action points

- Engage the whole organisation in developing an action plan.
- Review training of recruiters and ensure they are alert to diversity issues.
- Review and establish rigorous monitoring arrangements for all appointments.
- Review effectiveness and action to development opportunities including interorganisational mobility.
- Establish alliances with community groups, involving patients and wider community.
- Fast-track development programme for suitable individuals.

How and why is the trust's disability profile significant in providing quality clinical care to all sections of the community

- The disability issue is far wider than just physical access.

- There are different views on what the issue is. There is a need to understand how disabled staff feel and what is seen as discrimination by staff, patients and wider community.
- Need to avoid possible stereotyping which may occur through disabled/non-disabled categorisation. Needs of individual staff have to be met to allow their talents to emerge.

Action points

- There is a need for greater understanding of the difficulties encountered by disabled staff before solutions can be identified. Focus groups are a good way of approaching this.
- Local groups may be involved via visits to understand further the outcome of the audit.

A framework for change

Application 9:3

Christine Edwards, Susan McLaren,
Olive Robinson, Margaret Whittock

Part-time working in the nursing profession

Managing change: diversity, the key to success

INTRODUCTION

Currently, registered nurses comprise 56% of the NHS workforce, forming its most expensive professional group (Lane 1999, Pearce 1999). As the impact of skill shortages and elder care begins to take effect, managers are under pressure to ensure that they are appropriately skilled and flexibly deployed to deliver high-cost quality care. A diminishing supply of registered nurses coupled with high turnover rates (Gray 1997) ensures the centrality of flexible working to NHS strategy. This can:

- improve recruitment/retention levels of experienced trained nurses by permitting working parents to spend time with families
- mean less work-based stress, lower levels of absenteeism, lower recruitment costs for employers and higher morale generally
- promote cost-effective use of labour, allowing employers to match part-time hours to specific organisational requirements, avoiding expensive overtime and unsocial hours payments
- ensure compliance with the law with regard to the implementation of the Sex Discrimination Act, the European Union Part-time Work Directive and the Disability Discrimination Act.

Advantages to employers have been based on the experience of using part-time (PT) labour within a narrow range of female-dominated industrial sectors where conditions have been dictated by employer needs and are inferior to those of full-timers (FT). The characteristics of 'new' part-time work emerging in areas such as nursing are significantly different. Most part-time nurses have moved from full-time to part-time work within the same job, their requests often instigated by the need to accommodate caring commitments (Edwards & Robinson 1998).

The project

The Part-time Working in Nursing Project, collaboratively funded by the South East London Trust Education Consortium and the Equal Opportunities Unit of the NHS, examined these issues further, utilising results from a 1999–2000 cross-sectional survey of managers (n=51) and qualified full- and part-time nurses (n=386) from three outer London trusts (mental, acute and community). Part-time nurses accounted for 32% of those surveyed. Data were produced by a structured self-completion questionnaire with some semi-structured responses. The project aimed to identify the benefits, disadvantages and costs associated with part-time working from both management and employee perspectives.

ADVANTAGES AND DISADVANTAGES OF PART-TIME NURSING: PRELIMINARY RESULTS

Why do nurses work part time?

Of the female working population, approximately 45% work part time, particularly in female-dominated industries such as retailing where 70% of women are thus employed. Typically, such workers are used for jobs which do not require full-time hours, to cope with peaks and troughs in service demand and to avoid expensive overtime payments. Part-time working has been less common in nursing and is not part of a deliberate labour strategy aimed at cost saving. Rather, it aims to retain staff at a time of high labour turnover and staff shortages and is a reactive response by management to requests from full-timers to work part time, often to accommodate caring commitments.

- PTs (73%) are more likely than FTs (34%) to have children under 18 (p=0.000).
- 59% of PTs work part-time for childcare reasons.
- 14% of PTs have disabled/elderly dependants.
- 53% of all nurses thought it was either quite difficult or very difficult to combine caring responsibilities with employment. The majority of these were part time.

How do managers deploy their part-time staff?

Nurses' personal circumstances can be unpredictable and difficult to plan for. Consequently, managers often have little control over the ratio of part-timers to full-timers in their ward or department. Although managers surveyed needed to reduce costs, they did not appear to have designed jobs or recruited specifically to secure the

Part-time working in the nursing profession

cost savings benefits of part-time working despite significant variations in service demand.

- Only 16% of managers said they deployed staff to posts suitable for PT working.
- 64% said they deployed PTs in the same way as FTs.

Staff are not recruited directly to carry out roles or tasks uniquely suited to part-time working or to alleviate particular skills shortages. The main response to staff shortages was to retrain.

- 36% of managers were training/retraining existing staff.
- 22% were advertising a specific PT post.
- 22% were advertising 'flexible working' options.
- 64% of managers had no special measures to recruit women returners.
- Only 28% of PTs were recruited directly to PT jobs.

Most part-timers surveyed had returned to their existing full-time jobs on a part-time basis following maternity leave or other breaks, with few recruited directly to part-time jobs. Thus, management fails to capitalise on the labour cost reductions of flexible working which can be associated with these.

Advantages and disadvantages to management

Few managers (8%) regard part-time working as having no advantages. The main business case is seen to be the retention and recruitment of trained and experienced staff with over a third of managers believing they could deploy part-timers in order to cover peaks in service demand. Forty-two percent regarded part-time staff as being less stressed in what can be a traumatic work environment, leading to less absence and more flexible and enthusiastic staff (Box 9.3.1).

Managers were also candid about the disadvantages of part-time employment, with only 16% believing there were none (Box 9.3.2).

Box 9.3.1 Advantages of PT working to management in all three trusts (%) (n=51 managers)

Retention	62	Less absenteeism	30
Retains mature staff	54	More experienced	24
Recruitment	50	More flexible	24
Less stressed	42	More enthusiastic	14
Retains staff with family experience	40	Better quality of work	12
Covers peaks in service demand	36	More creative	10
Does jobs not requiring FT staffing	32	None	8

Box 9.3.2 Disadvantages of PT working to management in all three trusts (%) (n=51 managers)			
Problems giving & receiving info	40	Increased admin.	16
Not wanting unsocial shifts	28	Communication with staff	16
Continuity of service	28	Do not want responsibility	16
Communication with team	26	Increased costs	14
Problems completing tasks	26	Difficult to fit in with FT	12
Increased managerial time	24	working	
Do not want to tackle new tasks/roles	20	Communication with patient's family	10
		Communication with supervisors	10
Supervision more difficult	18	Other	16
None	16		

Problems with giving and receiving information appear common. Communication between colleagues, with management, supervisors and service users can be hindered by reduced presence in the workplace, hampering the flow of critical information gathering and impeding the performance of part-time staff. Part-timers may not integrate into a team if their shift patterns differ, if they work fewer hours or do not engage in informal events which support team building. Relationships may suffer where management fails to compensate the team for a reduced contribution by part-time members.

- 14% of mangers thought that PT working meant increased work for FT staff.
- 14% felt it led to feelings of inequity.
- 8% thought that FT staff were left with unpopular jobs.

Nursing services are provided on a 24-hour basis and part-timers are expected to undertake their share of the full range of associated duties. However, since most have caring responsibilities they find that irregular shift patterns and the unpredictable demands of the job present particular difficulties for family life. Attempting to fit part-timers into such a system can prove difficult, particularly if they are unwilling to cover shifts where managers feel they could most usefully be deployed. The fact that some part-timers seemed unwilling to tackle new tasks or roles, or accept responsibility, adds to resentment felt by full-time colleagues. Coupled with unwillingness to undertake overtime or rest day work, part-timers may not be the flexible labour resource they are believed to be and appear less likely than full-timers to carry out unpaid overtime.

- 48% of FTs as opposed to 33% of PTs worked additional hours in the previous week (p=0.010).

Part-time working in the nursing profession

223

- 20% of managers said they use unpaid overtime to deal with peaks in service demand.

While typical part-time work is determined by managers' assessments of service requirements, here, patterns are determined by negotiation between part-timers, line managers and a range of individuals. Survey data indicated no central policy in any of the trusts designed to deal with this.

The effects of part-time working on nurses

Whilst retaining skilled staff, managers are underutilising the resource by marginalising part-timers, risking serious skills attenuation by restricting opportunities for training and development. Many nurses complained about reduced responsibilities and status accompanying part-time work. Some managers resolve the problems outlined above by placing part-timers away from central roles and functions, either to accommodate their preferred pattern of work or because the function is deemed unsuitable for part-time work.

- 12% of managers think that posts of responsibility are unsuitable for PTs.
- 16% think posts requiring continuity are unsuitable.
- 6% think supervisory roles are unsuitable.
- 10% think mentoring roles unsuitable.
- 14% think that PTs should not have responsibility for a named patient.
- In allocating tasks and duties to PTs, 10% of managers reduced their range of tasks; 8% put them in less central roles, 6% reduced their responsibilities.

Some managers cited low status positions such as ward clerk as being suitable for part-time staff. Eight percent of part-timers had experienced a drop in grade on moving from full-time work or moved to less congenial duties to accommodate desired hours and shifts. Although part-timers are often older and more experienced than full-timers, some maintain that they are less involved across a range of responsible positions, have less opportunity to practise and develop skills and to gain the experience necessary for promotion. And, engagement in CPD is a requirement for continuing registration with the UKCC.

- 29% of FTs do higher grade work on a daily basis as opposed to 20% of PTs (no significant difference).
- 65% of FTs act as team leader at least once a month, as opposed to 48% of PTs ($p=0.003$) (chi square test).
- 47% of FTs act in place of a manager at least once a month, as opposed to 26% of PTs ($p=0.000$) (chi square test).

- 78% of FTs take charge of an area at least once a month, in comparison to 65% of PTs (no significant difference).
- 59% of FTs act as a clinical supervisor at least once a month, in comparison to 41% of PTs.
- FTs (53%) are more likely than PTs (40%) to participate in the development of clinical guidelines (p=0.013).

Part-timers' dissatisfaction with opportunities to learn new skills and with involvement in the decision-making process suggests an underutilisation of expensive, highly trained employees.

- FTs (56%) are more likely than PTs (39%) to attend management meetings (p=0.004).
- FTs (42%) are more likely than PTs (24%) to attend practice development meetings (p=0.004).
- FTs (25%) are more likely than PTs (14%) to attend research meetings (p=0.049).

Although there are policies of equal access to training for part-timers, their implementation appears uneven. Indeed, 34% of managers made no special arrangements to include part-time staff in the provision of training, and 12% gave priority to full-timers.

- 42% of PTs thought management neither encouraged nor discouraged training.
- 25% of PTs thought management encouraged training a lot.
- 68% of FTs have had some form of postbasic training in comparison to 61% of PTs (no significant difference).
- FTs (63%) are very satisfied or satisfied with their opportunities to gain qualifications, in comparison to PTs (48%) (p=0.022).

The picture, however, was not one of total dissatisfaction. Part-timers regarded the greatest advantage of part-time employment as allowing time for childcare and families, although the downside was the accompanying drop in salary. Such factors, coupled with lower levels of stress, sustained the quality of part-timers' lives generally, with a number expressing satisfaction in other areas.

- 70% of PTs believe that PT employment provides them with the opportunity to work the hours they want.
- Over 70% are satisfied with the continuity of care they offer and their ability to see tasks through to completion.
- 58% are satisfied with relationships with colleagues.

Nonetheless, part-timers expressed lower levels of satisfaction with the scope of their roles generally. Besides limiting promotional advancement, reduced experience of key operational duties leaves many ill equipped to compete with full-time colleagues. As a result of the factors outlined above, over twice as many part-timers (19%) as full-timers (8%) planned to be in a non-nursing job in 3 years' time.

Part-time working in the nursing profession

CONCLUSION

In short, while the survey suggests that part-time working can improve the quality of life for those involved, it may also lead to deskilling, thus adversely affecting the career development and promotion prospects of part-time nursing staff. And, although managers recognised the positive elements of part-time working, such as reduced stress levels, they were inclined to devalue part-timers, placing them away from central roles. Such action only succeeds in eroding the value of employers' retention strategies.

Currently, banks and agencies continue to be used by managers to deal with uneven peaks in demand, providing the flexibility that part-time nursing cannot. However, the demand for part-time employment opportunities, for women and men, will continue to rise. And while some nurses have found that part-time working accommodates their domestic commitments, there is still some distance to go before a balance can be struck between the costs and benefits of part-time working. As evidence from the survey indicates, systems of work will require considerable modification in order to deploy efficiently this 'new' diverse workforce.

References

Edwards C, Robinson O 1998 Better part-time jobs? A study of part-time work in two essential services. Kingston University, Kingston

Gray M 1997 Staying power. Nursing Standard 12(2):16–17

Lane N 1999 Sources of career disadvantage in nursing. Journal of Management in Medicine 13(6):373–389

Pearce L 1999 Cheap at the price. Nursing Standard 14(8):24–25

Managing change: diversity, the key to success

DEVELOPING THE DIVERSE WORKFORCE

Chapter **Ten**

Developing individuals

Janet Knowles

OVERVIEW

The aim of this chapter is to provide some understanding of differences in people, to identify ways of exploring these and approaching these differences positively as a source of strength and energy.

The chapter begins by focusing on the reasons for the unavoidable differences between human beings and points out that to understand others, we first have to understand as much about ourselves as possible. To assist the reader to consider this, a series of personal areas are identified and suggestions made about how best to gather the necessary data. Management skills are explored in this context and a questionnaire with accompanying 'useful tips' is supplied.

Objectives

This chapter explores the following themes and issues:

- the reasons for personal differences
- the importance of interpersonal perception
- the crucial need for using valid information rather than assumptions
- a structure for personal development
- managing a diverse workforce
- core management skills
- individual responsibility.

RECOGNISING AND ADDRESSING INDIVIDUAL NEEDS

Uniqueness is synonymous with being a human being; every person has an individual collection of characteristics that results in them being what they are. Let us initially consider some of the reasons for this enormous variety.

At birth each human baby is born into this world with a definitive set of genetic characteristics. The significance of the resulting inborn biases has been at the centre of the hereditary versus environment debate for over 60 years. The most recent research asserts that babies come into this world with certain 'preexisting conceptions' (Spelke 1991) that can shape the processes after birth through genetic programming. 'As each child becomes exposed to the process of maturation then although the sequential pattern is universally similar it is also agreed that experience has some effect.' The ongoing process of bonding and awareness opens up the response of one human being to another. This 'cocktail' of differences coming from genetics, family background, position in the family, culture, family trauma, social standing and wealth, to mention just a few factors, produces such a diverse population that the amazing thing is that we coexist as well as we do.

What we need to do, however, is to appreciate ways of understanding the 'shape' of individuals with a view to working more closely and effectively together as it is clear that whenever conflict or frustration interfere adversely with our working relationships, we are wasting both physical and mental energy.

To enable us to be aware of the reasons for the behaviour of others we first need to understand ourselves. This might be an area that you have already explored but for those who have not, it could turn out to be a life-changing experience.

The main areas to explore are:

- our personality, which gives some insight into our preferences and hence how we differ from one another
- our personal values, which can offer some understanding of the reasons for our attitudes towards people and things.

Studies have explored the stability of personality (McCrae & John 1992) and current thinking is that there are five domains of personality that can provide a comprehensive description of preferences and that these remain relatively stable in adulthood. These are:

- extraversion, with desirable traits of being outgoing, sociable and assertive

Developing the diverse workforce

- agreeableness, with desirable traits of kindness, warmth and trust
- conscientiousness, with desirable traits of organisation, thoroughness and tidiness
- emotional stability, with desirable traits of calmness, being even tempered and being imperturbable
- intellect or openness, with desirable traits of imagination, intelligence and creativity.

Values or beliefs are the enduring principles that govern the behaviour of individuals and considering our own values can enable us to understand that just as some behaviours and solutions are important to us, they are also unique. To others, your approach can seem to be inappropriate and confusing as they are using their own unique personal values as their basis of assessment. Our values provide us with 'comfort zones' so that when we are behaving in line with our values we feel energised and motivated and believe we are working well, whereas if we have to behave in ways that are not aligned to our values, we soon feel frustrated or lacklustre. This can be very energy absorbing and so the person involved can appear to be sluggish, reluctant or even lazy.

It is not only our raw perception of the behaviour of others that is important. We all judge each other on that basis but if you wish to get beneath the surface on a particular issue then you have to use our understanding of differences and how they can be utilised to achieve a beneficial outcome. The behaviour and approach of others are also the product of their unique blend of personal and environmental influences. It cannot be expected that these are in line with our own as even in childhood we tend to recreate the pattern which is familiar to us.

> What is rejection to one child is benign to another. What is warmth to a second child is confusing or ambiguous to another. For example, a child approaches another and asks to play. Turned down. The child goes off and sulks in a corner. A second child receiving the same negative reaction skips on to another partner and successfully engages him in play. Their experiences of rejection are vastly different. Each receives confirmation of quite different working models. (Sroufe 1988)

The background of prejudice and discrimination grows from our attitude towards our behavioural norms. Prejudice can be defined as a set of attitudes which cause, support and justify discrimination, i.e. an emotionally rigid attitude or predisposition in response to a group of people. Discrimination is the acting out of prejudicial beliefs, which can originate from the desire to maintain one's privileges or power in a particular situation. The mechanisms

Developing individuals

for the actions connected to prejudice are negative stereotypes, which result in avoidance. The mechanisms for discrimination are laws and norms, which result in mistreatment and unkindness. We are all susceptible to the effect that our assumptions have on our approach and the way in which we assess and respond to situations. Assumptions are fed by the information that we have already collected and stored throughout our lives. These assumptions nearly always outweigh observations and although this power to predict how situations are going to proceed and individuals behave can be very useful for moving things forward, it can also be detrimental to further realistic progress if the assumptions are wrong. If we are quick to assume rather than check on the facts then we run the risk of stopping and even damaging things for the future smooth running of situations. This is especially true if the assumptions are made about people and your expectations of them.

Try the small exercise in Box 10.1 to check on how you fit in with this scenario.

Box 10.1

Step 1
Choose someone new in your work environment whom you do not know very well.

Step 2
Observe this person closely and make some notes on the actual facts that you can verify, such as appearance, expressions, behaviour in some incidents and so on. In this case you are looking for the facts that cannot be disputed; for example, height, style of dress or attributes such as 'she is tall' or 'he is clumsy' rather than a subjective observation. It can be quite difficult to decide what is pure fact and what is subjective but perhaps you can help to clarify it for yourself by asking 'What is a given or verifiable piece of information in this particular situation?'.

Step 3
Then make another list but this time of your own assumptions about this person. This can include assumptions from what you have observed but mainly guesses and predictions about what you expect of this person based on your own attitudes and values. This can include religious likes or dislikes, opinions, etc. Some of these assumptions may be quite safe; for example, if she is tall then you might assume that she finds that her choice of clothes is restricted. However, some assumptions might be more debatable such as that she does not like being tall or that she deliberately avoids talking to small men. To get the best out of this exercise, be brutally honest with yourself and list all the assumptions that come to mind.

Box 10.1   Cont'd

Step 4
Having completed this exercise, estimate how many of these are correct. If possible, check out with the person themselves if you can explain the purpose of the exercise and possibly make a new friend or contact. If you consider that you could hurt the relationship at an early stage then ask another person who has a similar contact with them to write their assumptions and compare the lists.

Step 5
1. What did you learn about the initial collection of facts? Were they helpful in helping you to understand the person more?
2. Did this exercise provide some insight into how you make assumptions about people?
3. Does this now throw some light on how you perceive people and situations and the sort of information that you use to do that?

The point of this exercise is to encourage you to improve your observation of the salient facts about other people and situations and to enable you to form opinions on realistic and genuine data. Perceptions can be changed.

If we now turn to the development of all the workforce we can appreciate that in addition to all these personal needs that originate from existing differences, the nurse manager has an interesting and thought-provoking task ahead. Not only are the global needs of the vast organisation of the NHS and its patients to be addressed but also the aspirations and concerns of the individuals in their team.

DEVELOPMENT OF INDIVIDUALS

Before any real development can occur it is vital that the individuals concerned have a realistic understanding of their own strengths and range of expertise. This can prove to be a valuable exercise as it also motivates and encourages ownership of the process. Included in this audit are all the aspects of the following.

- Personality, which provides preferences.
- Values, which explores attitudes.
- Skills, which indicate specific abilities that can be generalised across situations.
- Experience, which provides proof of compatibility with a working environment.
- Achievements, which identify motivational incidents.
- Aspirations, which clarify future expectations.

233

This exercise provides a useful basis for determining individual strengths and future needs. By comparing aspirations and the present state of skills, development needs can be accurately assessed.

At this time it may be that particular aspects of inequality of every type – gender, race, disability and so on – can also be discussed and explored. The existing traditional hierarchical structure of the NHS has resulted in many areas of discrimination and now that these issues are firmly on the agenda, it provides us with an opportunity to start to build a discrimination-free workforce.

Skills development

A new era of skills development is being promoted by organisations that have thought strategically about needs in the future. Traditional approaches to equipping people for advanced skills and changing organisations and cultures have been evolved with a much greater emphasis on capability and personal skills. Recruitment of staff into many organisations, including the NHS, is not as dependent on established prejudices about gender, disability, race and status as it used to be although there is still need for improvement in some areas.

Management skills in a diverse workforce

As a manager of people it is important to explore the boundaries of your role and how you can best achieve success. This success depends on the way in which you facilitate the skills and strengths of the people with whom you work. This includes your subordinates, your peers and your bosses. With your subordinates you have the specific role of leader and manager, that of interpreting the larger issues into understandable and specific actions for others to complete. With your peers and superiors, the role becomes one of using negotiation and influence.

MANAGEMENT EFFECTIVENESS

What is management effectiveness? Can it be learned and how can it be maximised? What does a manger have to do to be perceived as being highly effective?

Managers on the whole wish to maximise their potential for growth and in order to grow as a manager, an individual must reach an understanding of how their behaviour in the management role affects competence. The following questionnaire will help you to gain an insight into your individual behaviour. It is based on the following assumptions about the management role; read through these and evaluate how much you agree with them.

- Managing means influencing the behaviour of others in order that they can contribute to the success, survival or growth of the organisation.
- The effectiveness of a manager is how successfully you influence the resultant performance (behaviour) of others with a wide range of different skills, experiences and backgrounds. Effectiveness is measured by the ability of a manager to combine the strengths of all these elements toward the achievement of organisational objectives. This includes how members of the working team reach their own objectives and value their work experience.
- One of the most important roles of a manager is to increase the probability that subordinates are successful in performing their jobs. This means that the effectiveness of a manager can depend on someone else's behaviour, that the actions of one person affect the success of another.
- There is a mutual dependency between the manager and the subordinate, each party needing the other to be effective in their respective jobs.
- The degree to which an effective manager influences the performance and satisfaction of a team member is largely a function of a manager's day-to-day management practices. It is not a function of personality, thoughts or attitudes; rather it is a function of behaviour – what is done and seen to be done.

Components of management effectiveness

Is there an ideal management profile? If so, what particular skills characterise it?

Research has been done by the Management Research Group (Mahoney & Rand 1985) to isolate specific criteria related to managerial effectiveness. This has included objective and subjective indices of productivity; ability to relate effectively to subordinates; skill in developing the talents and careers of employees and creating a work environment characterised by excellence; and the capability to accomplish relevant tasks.

Whilst it is obvious that managers in different functions possess specific and unique attributes, it was found that the same types of management behaviour are repeatedly associated with highly effective management across a variety of professional areas. These

Developing individuals

management behaviours are called the 'core sets' and comprise the following.

- Communication skills.
- The need to achieve objectives through other people and having regard and sensitivity for personal aspirations and need.
- Credibility in the eyes of staff.
- Sensitivity to people issues combined with critical management skills.
- Control and follow-up.
- Feedback.

The following questions were designed to allow each individual to consider their own specific management needs and, having identified strengths and areas for development, to be able to set up an individual action plan and use these criteria for planning a more effective approach.

Communication skills

1. How do you decide what and how much information you are going to disseminate to your subordinates?
2. How do you prefer to run meetings? Are you pleased with their effectiveness?
3. How do you know that any information that you have passed on has been received with the same meaning as you have given it?
4. How would you rate your listening skills?
5. Do you make time to talk to every member of your team on a regular basis?
6. How do you monitor the flow of information within a department?
7. How would you rate your persuasion skills?
8. How would other members of your team perceive your communication style?
9. Would you say that the meetings you run are focused?
10. Is there too much talk and not enough action in the team in your estimation?

Some useful tips

1. Find out what colleagues want to know rather than tell them what you think they should know.
2. Encourage your staff to share information.
3. Hold some meetings that do not have an agenda but are for the purpose of informal communication.

4. Make sure that you keep key people informed.
5. Talk openly with peers or people in other departments about 'communication breakdowns'. Devise ways to avoid them.
6. Return phone calls promptly.
7. At the end of the day, ask yourself what occurred that should be reported to other people.
8. Be aware of the messages that you send informally.
9. Focus your attention on understanding someone's meaning instead of formulating your response.
10. Ask open-ended questions to draw out a person's true thoughts and feelings by using phrases beginning with 'what', 'how', 'describe', 'explain', etc.
11. Look and be interested.
12. Avoid interrupting other people; wait until they have finished making their point.

Management focus

1. How much do you enjoy the management role?
2. Are you willing to take the responsibility for decisions?
3. Would you rather have a 'hands-on' approach than delegate?
4. Do you face up to conflict with assertiveness?
5. How much do you consider facing up to conflict to be a part of management?
6. Do you think that you understand management issues?
7. How would you describe your management style?
8. Are you willing to take responsibility for the actions of your staff?
9. How do you deal with poor quality of work in subordinates?
10. Do you capitalise on the status of being a manager?

Some useful tips

1. Start to see yourself as a leader and expect others to look to you for direction.
2. Visualise exactly how you would like to see the outcome of a project and think how others could achieve these outcomes.
3. Make it your business to know something about the lives of your staff and their concerns so that there is some evidence of your interest in them.
4. Show initiative in the face of difficulty, not by being authoritarian but by letting people know that you have the strength to follow through on a difficult assignment.

5. See yourself as the energiser for the group to build enthusiasm.
6. Become less self-conscious in your communication. Let others see you as a real contributor to the growth of the group.
7. Develop your decision-making expertise and allow others to see you doing it.
8. Be willing to make statements you stand by and be open with commitments and deadlines.
9. Learn to be tolerant of the mistakes and ideas of others.
10. Establish some goals that are innovative and look for more creative solutions than those normally used.
11. Recognise that your own future promotions will probably depend on your success in getting your people to take on more responsibility successfully.
12. Recognise that growth and jobs have ups and downs. There must always be some balance between structure and the allowance for individual initiative. As the individual shows ability to handle increasing responsibility, a decreasing amount of structure is needed.

Getting results

1. Do you think that you are seen to be credible in making demands, as there is evidence that the performance of a group is directly tied to the level of expectations of the leader?
2. Would you describe yourself as a results-oriented manager?
3. Do you feel that you are sometimes taken advantage of by your subordinates?
4. Do you consider it part of your managerial role to help to develop members of your team?
5. Are you sympathetic to people problems?
6. Do you think that you are perceived as being demanding?
7. How effective are your quality controls?
8. Do you set standards that are too high?
9. Is motivation of staff a problem for you? What do you think is the most effective way to do this?
10. Do you consider that you have done as much as possible to achieve a discrimination-free working environment?

Some useful tips

1. Establish the connection between the performance of the individual and the performance of the group, so that the ownership of success is shared and celebrated.

2. Have a member of your team write down their accountability and you do likewise separately, then have a meeting and compare notes. You might be surprised.
3. Become more aware of how you make assumptions and decisions in your everyday life and practise being more decisive.
4. Identify areas where each of your staff lacks confidence and work to overcome this confidence issue.
5. Develop a spirit of healthy competition between yours and other teams.
6. Explain how larger objectives can be broken down into smaller ones and put in sequential order, provide recognition when smaller objectives have been attained and design rewards appropriate to the situation and the person.
7. Develop an achievement-based culture, so that people are recognised for the effort they put in.
8. Recognise that any manager will be unpopular at times because of the demands they make and be willing to justify the demands you have made and accept criticism.
9. Accept your human limitations when carrying out complex tasks.
10. Ask members of your team to consider their own performance critically and come up with development plans.
11. Set goals that are stretching but obtainable and include the group in the setting of goals.
12. Make sure that there is time set aside for group interaction that is not directly involved with performance standards.

People

1. How important do you think your role is in achieving the goals of the function/organisation as a whole?
2. Can you be sympathetic without becoming too involved with the problems of your staff?
3. Do you find there is sometimes conflict between demanding high productivity and personal empathy?
4. Do your subordinates take advantage of your sympathy?
5. Are you perceived as being scrupulously fair?
6. Does your interactive style cause others to resist your requests?
7. Are you willing to listen to the views of your staff and respond realistically to their ideas?
8. Do your subordinates have confidence in your support of them?
9. How do you think your approach to the management of conflict is perceived by your subordinates?

Developing individuals

239

Six Steps to **Effective Management**

10. Are you able to balance the need to delegate with a real empathy with people?

Some useful tips

1. Provide adequate formal and informal channels to allow uncensored information to reach you.
2. Make a determined effort to empathise with a peer who has experienced a problem or suffered a disappointment.
3. Let your staff see you as a person with emotions. Share your feelings and ideas as this helps to develop trust.
4. Strengthen your ability to receive suggestions, including criticism, from a variety of sources. Do not avoid admitting you were wrong sometimes.
5. Cultivate your ability to be an active listener; paraphrase what you have just heard to be sure that you understood the communicator correctly.
6. Make sure you give people the chance to be heard without interrupting.
7. Learn to respect the reasoned argument of another, even if you disagree with it.
8. Establish a list of competencies that need to be developed in your group and see yourself as a facilitator of effective performance rather than as a final authority. Analyse what you are really trying to achieve – getting your staff to jump at your command or getting them to really perform.
9. Consider the negative effect of too much covert or overt conflict.
10. Recognising the emotional aspects of management as a sympathetic approach to your staff will increase performance.
11. Set up programmes that will stimulate a number of positive emotions: enthusiasm, confidence, fun, satisfaction, group cohesion and belonging.
12. Develop more confidence in yourself as a communicator and practise both on and off the job. Practise different communication approaches.

Control

1. How important is it for you to follow up delegated assignments?
2. Would you say that you run a highly disciplined unit?
3. Are you comfortable delegating important jobs to colleagues?

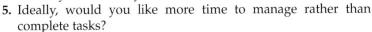
4. Would you describe yourself as detail conscious?
5. Ideally, would you like more time to manage rather than complete tasks?
6. Are you perceived as a 'hands-on' manager?
7. Do you pride youself on fostering innovation?
8. Are your staff sometimes confused by priorities?
9. Is completion of projects on time sometimes difficult to achieve and how do you ensure that this takes place?
10. Do your subordinates feel able to ask for help with their work without feeling a failure? How do you respond to appeals for help?

Some useful tips

1. Give broad-based responsibilities. Outline the result that you wish but allow the person to show some initiative if possible.
2. Don't act like a parent to your team; they need to learn for themselves as well.
3. Analyse the main recurring problems. Think about how these can be handled on a routine basis and if you do not know, either learn or get someone who knows how.
4. Perhaps you can set up a flowchart of department accountabilities and see how this relates to other departments.
5. Jointly set specific progress and target dates for assignments.
6. Communicate important action points in writing to all members of the team after meetings.
7. Institute a definite system for reminding people when an assignment has come due.
8. Incorporate the expectations of your boss into the performance expectations of your subordinates.
9. Identify the training needs of your team to close up the gaps between present expectations and actual performance, both individually and as a group.
10. Avoid becoming immersed in bureaucracy and prioritise your own work schedule according to effectiveness.

Feedback

1. How conscious are you of giving regular realistic feedback to your team?
2. Would you say that your subordinates know where they stand?
3. Are you known for promoting a positive environment?

Developing individuals

Six Steps to **Effective Management**

4. Do you find it difficult to give negative feedback?
5. Does your feedback style result in conflict or resentment?
6. Do you consider your assertiveness skills to be effective?
7. How would you like to modify your style to obtain results in line with your goals?
8. Do you invite realistic feedback of your performance and approach from your staff?
9. How do you prepare to give bad news to your subordinates?
10. Whose responsibility do you consider it to be to ensure that development of staff takes place?

Some useful tips

1. Make sure you balance the feedback in favour of the positive.
2. Share good news with your team.
3. Make praise part of the culture, not the exception.
4. Periodically have your staff evaluate their job and suggest how it might be done more effectively.
5. Identify present developmental needs and allocate the appropriate resources.
6. Be available to discuss problems relating to continuous growth and development.
7. Make training objectives as formal and tough as other departmental objectives.
8. Be sure that your team knows exactly what the final product of the assignment is supposed to look like.
9. Focus any conflict on issues rather than personalities.
10. Do not always look on conflict as detrimental; it can lead to new ideas and understandings.
11. Give a subordinate who has experienced failure a chance to succeed as soon as possible.
12. Learn to recognise the support needed by subordinates that may be outside their control. Take responsibility yourself for these action items.

DEVELOPMENT TOOLS

Individual development of skills, both hard and soft, only works well when the person takes responsibility for their own development. It is vital that a detailed action plan is created with the help of the manager concerned and evidence provided of third-party views and perceptions. This enables individuals to put their own

Developing the diverse workforce

perceptions into context and to learn how they are perceived by colleagues. To maximise the effect of any development programme, both coaching and mentoring are being used increasingly by organisations that have a pressured and demanding change project on hand.

Coaching

Coaching is one of the most powerful tools to accelerate learning where individual and collective knowledge are the most valuable assets. The core principles of coaching will be more essential to successful management in the future. As higher levels of performance continue to be sought there is a need for additional learning arenas to be added to the traditional management methods.

Coaching skills introduced into work environments will deliver enhanced performance by increasing self-esteem and sense of ownership for all staff. A coaching management style has been found to transform the culture of organisations so that all levels of staff work more cohesively together (Locke & Latham 1984). Coaching enables people to move beyond self-imposed limitations by engaging all their areas of skill not only to assimilate knowledge but also to understand how to incorporate this into their personal style and be a catalyst for organisational development.

Coaching helps to:

- circumvent common obstacles to learning
- stimulate learning
- stimulate change
- incorporate an understanding of cultural issues and put them in context.

Mentoring

Developmental mentoring is rapidly becoming an essential part of the human resources toolkit. It focuses on helping the learner achieve personal growth and is both empowering and mutually beneficial to the mentor and the mentee. A formal scheme builds on the informal mentoring that occurs naturally and helps to prevent most of the problems associated with informal relationships, such as marginalisation of minorities.

Evidence has been found of how effective mentoring programmes can be in reducing racism and 'classism' in working groups (Larke et al 1989).

Developing individuals

243

Formal courses

Whatever you have decided to aim for in your career, it is imperative that you identify the most appropriate and beneficial courses for the acquisition of skills to provide you with the credibility and justification for your future career aspirations. Whenever the question of learning new skills or further enhancing existing areas of expertise arises, great care has to be taken about the choice and suitability of the curriculum and the teaching style. It is not uncommon for people to accumulate a variety of qualifications and then to discover that they have priced themselves out of the next feasible career step. Qualifications need to be matched with relevant experience. To avoid this it is wise to talk to members of staff or other experienced and knowledgeable people who can advise you about the suitability of particular paths of development.

For individuals to truly develop, the impetus has to originate within themselves. The process has to be one of targeted awareness of needs to achieve goals and aspirations. If it is your own personal development then you can stand back, assess where you are and where you would like to be in your career and/or lifestyle, but the goals have to be realistic. If you set goals that are unachievable then you are bound to fail and will then perceive yourself as a failure which is damaging to self-esteem and motivation. Move forward little by little and you will gain in confidence and maturity.

In helping others to develop, it is important to see yourself as a leader and gain satisfaction from their gain in skills and expertise. The best managers are those who have a reputation for assisting those around them to develop.

CONCLUSION

This chapter has explored the importance of and possible approaches to developing individuals within the NHS. Initially the reasons for diversity were discussed and the power of perception identified. The sources of personal differences were mentioned and how intentions could be misinterpreted by using subjective and invalid assumptions. It has been stressed throughout that the responsibility for personal growth lies with the individual and not with anyone else. Preparation for development is crucial and the relevant, accurate personal data have to be collected. The approach to this is outlined in the text.

The background to prejudice and discrimination was examined and the downside of allowing the reactions of other people to interfere with the objective consideration of fact mentioned. Management of people requires using personal strengths in different ways according to the context and their level of expertise. A core group of management skills was identified and checklists provided to enable readers to identify individual style. Management tips were also listed to give inexperienced managers some benchmarks for their behaviour.

Practice checklist

The following issues may help you to assimilate the learning from this chapter into everyday practice.

- The importance of making assumptions from a factual rather than an emotional basis.
- The ability to stand back and review the differences of your colleagues and how this affects their perception of each other and of you.
- Take a more strategic view of interpersonal relationships within your team and challenge yourself to facilitate effective interaction between them.
- Value diversity and consider positive ways of utilising the breadth of skills.

Discussion questions

As a member or perhaps a leader of a team, reflect upon what you have learned in this chapter and organise an action plan for yourself that will provide clear criteria of success for your activity.

- Have you addressed the motivation of your team and how best to energise the individuals, particularly in times of stress?
- Management of conflict is vital to good working relationships. What have you learned about your own approach that can help to achieve a positive environment?
- Comment upon your preferred approach to maintaining an effective and developing team, analyse the pitfalls and how you can overcome or work round them.

Developing individuals

References

Larke P, Wiseman D, Bradley C 1989 Cross-cultural mentoring: the impact of a cross-cultural mentoring relationship on attitudinal changes of teachers. Mentoring Resource Center, Baltimore

Locke E A, Latham G P 1984 Goal setting: a motivational technique that works. Prentice-Hall, Englewood Cliffs, NJ

McCrae R R, John O P 1992 An introduction to the five factor model and its applications. Journal of Personality 60:175–215

Mahoney J, Rand T 1985 Management effective analysis. Management Research Group, Portland, Maine

Spelke E S 1991 Physical knowledge in infancy. Reflections of Piaget's theory. In: Carey S, Gelman R (eds) The epigenesis of the mind. Essays on biology and cognition. Erlbaum, Hillsdale, NJ

Sroufe L A 1988 The role of infant care-giver attachment in development. In: Belsky J, Nezworski T (eds) Clinical implications of attachment. Lawrence Erlbaum, Hillsdale, NJ

Further reading

Brown A 1995 Organisational culture. Pitman Publishing, London

Kroeger O, Thuesen J M 1992 Type talk at work. Delacourt Press, New York

Woodcock M, Francis D 1982 The unblocked manager. Gower, Aldershot

Developing the diverse workforce

Application **10:1**

Barbara Burford

Positively Diverse: ensuring a workforce fit for purpose

POSITIVELY DIVERSE

The Department of Health is committed to equal opportunities and through its Equal Opportunities Unit has invested in organisations across the country through the Positively Diverse programme.

Positively Diverse started out as an organisational change programme aimed at developing the capacity to manage diversity in a Bradford NHS community trust to the benefit of the communities that it served. It is now a national programme, which is seen as an organisational development programme, a community of practice and a strategic framework.

The programme has created a network of national reference sites, working together as a community of practice to develop and model effective strategic planning and implementation aimed at widening access to the health and social care workforce from our local communities. A key strategic objective is to ensure that the workforce is equipped to deliver appropriate accessible services which tackle inequalities and are responsive to diversity.

The programme was originally developed at Bradford Community Health in 1995 as a response to the organisation's perception that it could no longer continue to talk about 'poor take-up of services' by local minority groups but rather had to reframe the issue as (for whatever reason) *'poor provision of services'*. In 1997 the NHS Equal Opportunities Unit commissioned further development of Positively Diverse and the programme is now working with more than 40 organisations. The national reference group organisations chosen exhibited the following characteristics:

- there is coverage of all regions and all types of health care organisation
- a large number of the organisations serve populations with greater than 10% of people from minority ethnic groups

- there is coverage of some of the five most underprivileged estates
- there is involvement of all the 'players' in at least two health action zones
- at least one trust has a large Private Finance Initiative in progress or imminent.

The programme also gains from the experience and involvement of university faculties, schools and colleges, the Commission for Racial Equality (CRE), racial equality councils, TECs and employment services.

Positively Diverse focuses on bringing about organisational change in equal opportunities practice and diversity management, using an action research model. The action research approach is used because it enables change and understanding to be pursued at the same time. The cyclical nature of the process, which involves action, review, critical reflection and planning, will enable creative and iconoclastic ideas, solutions and interventions to flourish by providing support and safety to minimise risk, as well as channelling robust theoretical and practical feedback and critique from an advisory group made up of HR directors, chief executives, senior nurses and professionals and other stakeholders.

Each organisation involved has appointed a project manager, reporting to board level, who will be responsible for and trained to deliver the programme locally. The programme is based around answering four questions.

Where are we?

This first stage holds up a mirror to the organisation, its relationships, processes, mechanisms and culture. A computerised audit, developed at Bradford and based on and extending the CRE racial equality standards to cover other areas of diversity, is performed. The results of this, plus other organisational data and community demographics, informs the next step.

Where do we want to go?

The implementation needs of the government's ambitious programmes for the NHS, as set out in the White Paper *The new NHS* and the Green Paper *Our healthier nation*, mean that each organisation must develop a detailed profile of the workforce capability, capacity and competencies necessary to deliver its new local agenda. Based on this profile and using the audit results to illuminate the gaps between where they are and where they need to be, the organisations will move to the next step.

How are we going to get there?

Action planning within each organisation will be able to draw upon:

- collective knowledge and insights available from other reference group sites
- interventions already developed and implemented through Positively Diverse in Bradford, for example, the Healthcare Apprenticeship Scheme (used as a national exemplar of how to recruit minority ethnic individuals into nursing) and the Jobshop, a joint initiative providing access to and advice about all health care jobs and professions
- a developing knowledge base of best practice and effective interventions within the NHS and externally
- growing links with the communities that they serve.

This will enable them to develop action plans and goals that model the crosscultural and crossorganisational ways in which we will seek to mainstream good equal opportunities practice and diversity management so that they become part of sound and beneficial business practice.

The aim of these plans will be to make diversity real in the workplace by concrete, properly implemented and evaluated policies, procedures and interventions and to develop and plan bridges and ladders for entry and progress into health care professions by underrepresented, socially excluded and marginalised groups.

How will we know that we have got there?

The detailed statistical and qualitative information delivered by the yearly rerun of the Positively Diverse audit will enable each organisation to evaluate the effectiveness of the work that it has undertaken.

The organisations will be able jointly and individually to engage in a period of review, reflection and further action planning as they seek to ensure that gains are consolidated and failures learnt from.

NATIONAL OUTPUTS

By the end of the first year, each organisation produces a gap analysis report, showing a picture of the organisation in the present, the goals and aspirations that it has set for the next year and the strategic direction it wants to follow and, most importantly, how it intends to bridge the gap.

These reports also demonstrate the ways in which these organisations will seek to develop a range of performance measures, both organisational and individual, and how to achieve and maintain high-level ownership and accountability, as well as ways of building equal opportunities and diversity management into each line manager's objectives.

A workforce fit for purpose

Using the data from these local audits, a national benchmark report will be produced. This will inform and support other NHS organisations wishing to audit themselves. The national reference group (NRG) sites will also begin to act as regional centres of expertise to support this work.

During the second year, when the NRG sites are implementing their action plans, there will be opportunities for further group, consortium and individual development and testing of new and reworked interventions.

The work, experiences and lessons learnt during this period will also be presented at a national conference. Because they are seeking to model the new NHS, the organisations involved will be readily available and informed sounding boards for future policy development and consultation processes.

A Positively Diverse knowledge base will be created, available in printed form and as a website. This will enable the swift dissemination of the products, insights, expertise and lessons learnt from the programme, thus enabling the whole service to build on the work already done and to save effort and resources by not starting from scratch each time.

Application **10:2**

Joy Foster

Networking: a personal view

Women in senior management positions are frequently isolated from other women. Even in the health and safety care sectors where women predominate in the workforce, women senior managers are usually in the minority in their management teams. They are confronted with difference. They are set apart from other managers as a result of their gender but they are also set apart from the majority of other women by virtue of their role and responsibilities. Within the organisation, they are likely to be distanced from other women by hierarchy. Outside the organisation, their success in reaching senior positions is likely to separate them from women peers along a number of dimensions. For example, in social settings the roles of wife and mother are often a source of shared experience for women yet many women managers remain single or child free. For women, sharing the experiences gained as managers with other women is likely to be difficult.

It has been noted (e.g. Davidson & Cooper 1992, Vinnicombe & Colwill 1995) that women are frequently excluded from the informal networks of organisations. Often these tend to be based on sporting activities such as football, cricket, squash or golf. Not only does this disadvantage women in excluding them from the informal exchange of information which takes place beyond the confines of meetings and office discussions but it denies them opportunities to explore issues or build relationships and it may deny them access to information about jobs. Often, too, women managers have not had experience of role models or mentors who are women and find themselves surrounded by models of managers who are men. The sexuality of organisations and women's visibility as women can result in their contacts being the subject of public scrutiny. All these factors can leave women senior managers very much on their own within their organisations.

Establishing networks specifically geared to facilitating the sharing of practice and experience is a practical way of developing contact with other women and helping to counter this exclusion. Sharing ideas, strategies and experiences can be very helpful not only in

251

increasing confidence and motivation but also in furthering strategic issues.

On a personal level, I have been fortunate in enjoying membership of AWSM, the Association of Women Senior Managers in Personal Social Services. The group grew out of a series of seminars to disseminate my own research findings during the course of my postgraduate degree. The group consists primarily of senior managers in social services departments but includes some from voluntary organisations and other public sector organisations. The network has been meeting for over 10 years on a quarterly basis and has succeeded in maintaining a flat network structure in a largely hierarchical world. It has organised conferences and seminars for a wider audience than its own membership and encouraged reflection on gender issues in service provision and delivery.

Not only do meetings provide an opportunity to reflect on current issues, to listen to a chosen speaker, to participate in personal development exercises and so on but, perhaps more importantly for myself on a personal level, they have enabled me to meet with other women whose values and experiences resonate with my own. Within this network it is safe to discuss ideas before they are fully thought through and to seek to develop them further and to share issues and concerns.

The network members have agonised repeatedly about our responsibilities to women elsewhere in the organisations. We are conscious of our privileged position as middle-class, predominantly middle-aged, educated and currently all white women. We would like to see this change and are concerned to increase our own diversity. Moreover, it never seems legitimate for women managers to take time to meet needs of our own and the pressures on women's time often make attendance difficult. To balance the focus on ourselves and to seek to be supportive of other women, the network has regularly organised conferences on women's issues. Repeatedly, we are surprised at the atmosphere in these conferences where there is little evidence of competitiveness or status consciousness but a real sense of empowerment for women through being with other women.

Several members have also established women's networks within their authorities or departments. Some of these have been initiated through training ventures for women, others more informally arise through, for example, setting aside a lunch hour on a monthly basis. If there are two or three women interested in meeting together a network can begin!

We have encountered the ambivalence of some women who feel that separateness is an inappropriate strategy or who are reluctant to be identified with 'women's issues' and the criticism of those who consider the group as elitist. Members have experienced the obstruction of some men hostile to their attendance and the respect of a few who are familiar with the issues. But we have also encountered the delight of women who see women prepared to identify themselves as powerful women concerned about their own and others' exclusion and the encouragement which comes from not always being in a minority.

References

Davidson M J, Cooper C L 1992 Shattering the glass ceiling: the woman manager. Paul Chapman, London

Vinnicombe S, Colwill N L 1995 The essence of women in management. Prentice Hall, London

Networking: a personal view

Section Five

THE DIVERSE TEAM – MAKING IT WORK

Chapter **Eleven**

The multiracial team: the challenges ahead

John James, Carol Baxter

O V E R V I E W

This chapter begins by arguing that the presence of black and ethnic minorities* in Britain has not resulted in a multiracial approach in the NHS, neither in terms of service delivery nor employment. In light of the current move to increase the numbers of black ethnic minority nurses, the challenges for managers in addressing this aspect of diversity are discussed with a particular focus on intergroup dynamics and racism awareness. Drawing on work carried out in the field of social work, the chapter concludes with an exploration of the particular position of black managers and relevant managerial

* There is no one word that embraces all members of minority racial groups in this country. At the same time, there are many people from ethnic minority communities in Britain who do not identify themselves as black but who, because of ethnic origin, language, cultural or religious differences, share a common experience of discrimination and inequality. No single term is completely acceptable to everyone. The use of both terms together, however, includes any individual who suffers the effects of racism. It is also recognised that for some people using the term is a compromise.

strategies for services in enabling them to assist the organisation to be more responsive to the needs from this section of the population.

INTRODUCTION

Cox (1991) distinguished between three types of organisations according to their attitudes towards diversity. *Monolithic* organisations are those which have a large majority of one demographic group (typically white males), especially in higher level positions. Women and minority group employees are expected to adopt to the norms and values of the majority group in order to survive. *Pluralistic* organisations are more mixed in composition. They take more steps to hire and promote minority group members but still expect women and minorities to adhere to the norms and values of the majority group. *Multicultural* organisations actively value diversity. They respond to employee differences by encouraging members of different cultural groups to adopt some of the norms and values of other groups. A multicultural approach promotes appreciation of differences associated with the heritage, characteristics and values of members of different groups as well as respecting the uniqueness of each.

The term *multicultural* is often used synonymously with another term – *multiracial*. These terms are not, of course, mutually exclusive but the former viewpoint has been criticised because it does not address the issue of racial discrimination or how it can be eradicated. Whereas the multicultural viewpoint tends to attribute inequalities in society to the cultural differences that exist between different communities in Britain and sees the solution in promoting greater understanding between cultures, the multiracial viewpoint acknowledges the fact that 'race' is one of the most significant factors contributing to unfair treatment and social inequalities in British society.

RACIAL INEQUALITIES IN HEALTH AND HEALTH CARE

Like a cosy image on a Christmas card, many would have us believe that black and ethnic minority groups, having been part of Britain for over a century, now live in a country where the boundaries between the races have been erased. Closer examination, however, suggests that whilst the boundaries persist, the arrival of black and ethnic minority groups into the UK during the 1950s and 1960s has helped in many ways to shape and design multicultural Britain. Thirty years later a culture that is distinctively black and British has emerged in the major cities in Britain. To some this may be regarded as 'street' culture but it is apparent in other areas such as the arts, fashion, music, law, journalism and sport.

The visible black presence in the NHS is largely a reflection of social engineering. Black people have been crucial to the NHS from its inception. In the early 1950s Britain found itself with a new and expanding health service which it could not afford to staff. In the wake of the post-war boom British people were reluctant to work long hours for low pay and this compounded the labour shortage. Before this period, hospitals had relied on Irish workers to make up shortages in both nursing and auxiliary categories. However, after the war the marked reduction of Irish immigrants meant that a new source of labour for the health service had to be found. It was to the Commonwealth that Britain turned for a cheap source of labour to provide the solution to the staffing problems. The recruitment campaigns for nurses were extensively and energetically pursued, senior British nurses visiting Commonwealth countries personally for this purpose. This scheme of nurse recruitment escaped the tight restrictions of the 1962 and 1965 Commonwealth Immigration Acts, which limited the number of unskilled workers allowed to enter Britain. Since immigration policy in Britain has always been determined by manpower needs, the NHS was less severely affected by immigration controls than most other sectors of the British economy and was able to receive a steady supply of student nurses from overseas. Subsequent employment measures such as section 11 funding in the aftermath of the riots in some black neighbourhoods in 1981 further accelerated the employment of black people into non-professional public sector jobs.

Despite the emergence of distinctly black British culture in the UK, the following section demonstrates that the presence of black and ethnic minority people in the NHS has had very little effect on the way services are delivered to this section of the population and the elimination of racial discrimination is a goal which the NHS is still struggling with (DoH 2000).

Health and health care experiences

It is well recognised that black and ethnic minority people experience worse health and health care than their white counterparts

(Acheson 1998). In terms of mortality, for example, deaths from coronary heart disease are nearly twice the national average amongst people from South Asian origin and all visible minority communities recorded higher rates of strokes than the white population (DoH 1992). In mental health services there is also substantial evidence that black people are more likely to be detained in locked wards of psychiatric hospitals and to be diagnosed schizophrenic and are less likely to receive psychotherapy than their white counterparts (Smage 1995).

A recent survey of 160 000 people throughout the European Union concluded that almost a third of Britons admit to being racist (European Commission 1999). This racism, which is deeply rooted in British culture, is also reflected in the NHS. The recent Stephen Lawrence inquiry has also ensured that public attention remains focused on racism in Britain (Macpherson 1999). The Lawrence Report not only charged the police with 'institutionalised' racism but effectively charged the rest of British society with collusion. It also prompted organisations in the public sector to admit that their organisations are institutionally racist, as detected in 'processes, attitudes and behaviour which amount to discrimination through unwitting prejudice, ignorance, thoughtlessness and racist stereotyping which disadvantage minority ethnic people' (Macpherson 1999).

Racial discrimination is evident in access, service delivery and employment practice and seriously affects the standard of care people from black and ethnic minorities receive and thus their confidence in using the NHS to its full potential (Royal College of Physicians 1993). The Secretary of State for Health recently initiated a full investigation into reports that donated organs were accepted by health trusts on condition that they did not go to a black person.

Employment experiences

The overall percentage of black and ethnic minority people in the workforce compares well with the working population as a whole.

Several reports, both historically and recently, point to the fact that the NHS has not been fully tapping the potential of this section of its workforce. They are frequently found in jobs which do not reflect their abilities and are undervalued by colleagues (CRE 1983). Black nurses are found working in the less attractive specialisms such as geriatrics, psychiatry, in hospitals for the mentally ill and the mentally handicapped and on night duty

(Beishon et al 1995, King's Fund 1990, Lee-Cunin 1989). There is a disproportionately large number of black and ethnic minority employees in ancillary and nursing auxiliary grades, as compared to the minute numbers and in some cases total absence of black employees at middle and top management levels within the NHS. In the 1980s the underrepresentation of women in senior, managerial and professional positions in the NHS prompted the establishment of a women's unit within the service whose task was in part to devise a remedial strategy to positively address the underrepresentation. This was essentially a form of affirmative action for women and it has been generally viewed as a successful initiative. Whether it has enabled women from black and ethnic minorities to attain senior positions is less clear.

However, in view of the poor experience of black people entering the NHS in the 1960s and 1970s, particularly in nursing, the number of young black people who now see the NHS as a successful career path has been falling. There is a particularly low percentage of Asian nurses and a low percentage of nurses in the younger age groups. Moreover, the changing demographic composition of the UK workforce has brought the potential labour supply for Britain's minority ethnic communities into sharper focus. The age profile of this section of the population is younger in comparison with the population as a whole; thus people born outside the UK represent a significant pool of potential young workers (OPCS 1993).

Experience of service delivery

It is recognised that if the NHS does not recruit and retain ethnic minorities it will, particularly in some areas of the country, increasingly be faced with severe shortages (see Application 2.1). Furthermore, if such groups are underrepresented in the nursing, midwifery and health visiting workforce, this undermines the potential of the NHS to provide appropriate services to this section of the population.

The presence of black and ethnic minorities in the NHS should be a positive step towards addressing the inequalities faced by this section of the population and should improve relations with diverse clientele. Because of their similar cultural and religious background, black and ethnic minority clients will be able to identify gaps in the service and other ways in which current provision is inadequate in a way that is not so easy for a white person to do. Ahmed (1980), in referring to social work practice, identified that

The multiracial team: the challenges ahead

black staff have found it necessary to develop their own appropriate models and patterns of practice which they feel more closely reflect the needs of individuals from their communities. Furthermore, experience in the field of learning disabilities demonstrated that employing staff who can communicate with people who do not speak English can and does result in a startling increase in service uptake by non-English speaking patients. Such impact will be even more important in the health setting, where the support and care required is of a personal and intimate nature.

THE MANAGEMENT OF THE MULTIRACIAL TEAM

In recognition of the potential contribution to the provision of effective, accessible and culturally appropriate services to the diverse communities, high-profile attention is currently being given to achieving a workforce drawn from all sections of society. Concern about the falling numbers of ethnic minority nurses in particular has lead to various national initiatives which specifically address their recruitment and retention: recent national and London-based recruitment campaigns were created to appeal to people from this section of the population. In anticipation of the imminent increase in the ethnic diversity of the nursing workforce, it is essential that managers develop strategies to ensure that past mistakes are not repeated and that staff are enabled to contribute to their true potential in making the service truly multicultural. Managers will need to develop their skills in bringing about cohesive output from multiracial teams and in particular how to get the additional value that black and ethnic minority people bring beyond their professional training and experiences. They will thus need to acknowledge and understand the emergence of black British culture and the relationship of that to the beliefs, values, norms and ground rules that define how this new emerging NHS will operate.

Intergroup dynamics

Skilful and effective management of diversity will require an appreciation of the complexities involved. The diverse outlook which is being pursued can also pose a dilemma for organisations since multicultural teams can be more prone to exhibit dysfunctional team processes. Kanter's classic work documents what happens to 'Os' (representing token members of a minority) when

The diverse team – making it work

they are in a team that has mostly 'Xs', whatever the basis for distinguishing between Xs and Os may be (Kanter 1977). Os tend to experience greater performance pressures than Xs. They risk being classified according to the stereotype of Os, whatever that stereotype may be. Also they tend to be excluded from informal activities in which Xs like to engage. These problems exist when a team is demographically imbalanced with respect to a notable characteristic such as race or gender. In the new NHS, a critical managerial task for managers is to create an environment that can adequately deal with these intergroup relations and dynamics.

Black and ethnic minority staff cannot produce to their maximum potential as long as they are managed with the traditional Euro-centric standard NHS techniques. Skills required in leading and directing people of many cultures in attaining organisational and personal goals have been discussed in Chapter 1. Additional management techniques that will take the issue not only of culture but of racism into account and which will thus support black and minority staff and capitalise on their potential are as follows.

- Feedback or input on minorities should be understood and probed. Managers should probe both negative and positive feedback on minority staff. It is important to test the validity of the feedback, which is one way of removing racism or sexism from the feedback/input.
- Minorities should be included in decision-making processes. It is vital that managers include minority staff early in any decision that will have a major impact on them. If they do not, assumptions made by white managers may be flawed or wrong. Health policy makers realise they need to involve black and ethnic minorities in drawing up service strategies and frameworks at local level but research has shown that work in this area requires development.

    Effective intercultural communication skills are thus a highly valued asset. As highlighted by McEnrue (1993), this includes characteristics such as: the capacity to accept the relativity of one's own knowledge and perceptions, to be non-judgemental, tolerance of ambiguity, respect for other people's ways, backgrounds, values and beliefs, empathy, flexibility, willingness to acquire new patterns of behaviour and belief and humility to acknowledge what one does not know (see Chapter 1).
- Like probing input and feedback, managers exploring black and ethnic minority individuals' perceptions, experiences and assumptions about a given situation will help mutual understanding.

The multiracial team: the challenges ahead

- An open and transparent style of interaction is particularly important when dealing with black and ethnic minority staff. Many people from black and ethnic minorities will have been the victims of racial discrimination and sexist behaviour. If that is so, they will naturally be suspicious of those white managers who do not interact within an open management style.
- Racist behaviour and the resultant anger and resentment of black people must be effectively managed by both whites and blacks. Black and minority staff will need support in managing anger arising from the racism of others. Equally, white managers must be able to prevent inappropriate racist behaviour in the manager/subordinate relationship.
- It is vital that a sensitive and skilful manager or mentor is selected for a new minority recruit to the organisation or team. This should facilitate early success.
- Training, coaching and action learning can help to develop reasonable managerial skills in this area.

Racism awareness

Racism awareness training was originally designed to help white people specifically to examine the roots of their own racism and how this is reflected in their social and work relationships and help them take responsibility for challenging this. This aspect of staff development has in recent years been submerged by a new focus on the wider issues of diversity.

It is being argued here, however, that racism awareness still has a significant role to play in the development of multiracial teams and that all staff (from both the majority and minority communities) will need to have an opportunity to reflect on the issue of racism. White staff will need assistance and support to unpack years of conditioning and embrace difference to create an environment free from negative discrimination. Black staff will need support to redefine themselves and their reality, instead of internalising white people's perception of them.

It is important to emphasise that, although there will be incidents of personal racism, most people in the caring professions take seriously their obligation to treat all people with respect and would regard deliberate, overt discrimination as unprofessional behaviour. Institutional racism is far more common and more damning. It can happen:

- by default, where the way things are done within organisations does not take account of the needs of black and ethnic minority people
- where the rules and regulations of the organisation apply equally to all, but they have the effect of excluding this section of the population while maintaining the privileged position of white people
- where people in positions of power base their decisions on assumptions and stereotypes.

An understanding of the historical power relationships between black and white people and the legacy this has left in society is important, as is understanding of the different values, expectations and ways of doing things of people of cultures other than their own. Here the difference in emphasis between multicultural and multiracial has important implications for the training of health professionals. For example, a multicultural approach to training would see as its purpose the focusing of attention on all groups represented in society – Irish, Greek, Cypriot, Welsh, Afro-Caribbean, Jewish, Scottish, Bengali – for the purpose of understanding their cultures. A multiracial approach to training, on the other hand, would focus in particular on the specific issues that arise from the areas of black/white relations and racial inequality. Such a programme would, of course, look at ethnic minority culture but from the viewpoint of understanding how white perceptions of minority cultures may contribute to inequality and disadvantage among those minorities.

Such awareness and knowledge by themselves can simply result in guilt, which will not work as a spur to action. Staff will be seeking inputs which they can immediately recognise as essential to their work. Thus, it is essential that the practical implications are addressed and that staff have an opportunity to identify and develop specific skills reflective of antiracist practice.

Thus the primary purpose of racism awareness training is the development of an informed, skilled, sensitive and competent practitioner who has a critical approach to the health and health care needs of this group of patients and who recognises and challenges the ethnocentric orientation of care provision.

Specific objectives will be to enable participants to:

- reflect on their own attitudes and beliefs, in order to develop ways of thinking about people which value their racial and cultural differences

The multiracial team: the challenges ahead

- increase their knowledge and understanding, through factual information about evidence of racial inequalities in health, variations in patterns of illness and differing cultural and linguistic norms
- acquire practical skills and competencies in delivering care to all client groups including those whose colour and culture may be different from their own
- develop ideas for achieving change; for example, building up networks through contact with others, sharing experiences and ideas and exchanging examples of good practice.

The basic premise and principles in racism awareness training are outlined in Box 11.1

Box 11.1 Basic premise and principles in Racism Awareness training

- Racism is part of the culture within British society and individuals within it have been socialised into this from childhood.
- Racism encompasses not only prejudice but also the power held by white society to translate its prejudices into practices that initiate and perpetuate injustice.
- Black and white people are hurt by racism in different ways. In becoming aware about our own racism the pain of that hurt must be made conscious.
- Racism Awareness training enables individuals to explore how racism is part of themselves, the organisations in which they work and in society as a whole.
- Participants are responsible for their own learning. The trainer acts primarily as a facilitator who helps to build a group sense of trust, understands that guilt can block change and is willing to confront racism and help individuals to make choices about future assumptions and behaviours.
- The trainer needs to have a deep knowledge and understanding of how racism operates, as well as skills as a group facilitator and sensitivity to group process and individual emotions.
- Racism Awareness does not take place in one-off short workshops. It is part of a broader programme of organisation development towards equality of opportunities in which the overall aim is to confront and change institutional structures and procedures.
- The ultimate value of Racism Awareness training lies in its generation of both individual and group commitment to action for changing racist practices and achieving justice. This is achieved by overcoming emotional blocks that can undermine other initiatives such as equal opportunity programmes or antiracist confrontations.

The diverse team – making it work

VALUING AND SUPPORTING BLACK MANAGERS

Much of the literature on modern management in the NHS fails to explore the impact of racism on the psychological and behavioural processes of black and minority staff in white settings and the movement or development that evolves as a result of those staff efforts to achieve success and equality of opportunity. Ahmed (1992), in her seminal work exploring the experiences of black managers working for white organisations, is one of the few sources located in the UK. Based on action research over a 2-year period with social work teams, this work revealed that black and ethnic minority managers:

● are often expected to demonstrate their ability to manage as defined by the white perception of management
● are expected to accept the white role models of management abilities and develop them accordingly
● often come under pressure to deny their ethnicity and be a manager first and black last (if at all).

And there is a common assumption that they:

● are less qualified, less experienced and less trained and thus less able than their white counterparts
● do not have any 'special' abilities which merit attention.

Ahmed's conclusions bear much relevance to the NHS where detailed work of this nature is yet to be conducted. It is therefore crucial that black managers have the opportunities for developing and realising their management abilities without having to disown their blackness, in the same way that white managers are not questioned about whether they are white first and manager second or vice versa. She states:

> Imagine a situation that could happen if white managers were ordered to leave their whiteness and genders outside their managerial roles. They would cease to function as human beings. No black person can build on their management abilities and develop as capable managers, if they are dehumanised by their or others' rejection of their very being, that is being Black.

Ahmed (1992) cites the following case study which points up some of the most pertinent issues that many black managers have to deal with and suggests that it highlights one of the most fundamental management issues – management accountability. She puts

The multiracial team: the challenges ahead

The diverse team – making it work

Case study

A project on monitoring the quantity and quality of service delivery to black and minority ethnic communities was jointly managed by a white and black manager. The project worker was black. A steering committee was set up with black and white members to overview the project and assist in making progress.

- The white manager's management agenda was that the project work needed to be organised in a way that was going to satisfy the funding agency, even if it meant watering down some of the findings, as they may be too controversial.
- The black manager's role was only to advise on 'race' aspects of the project as and when felt necessary and appropriate.
- The project worker directly reported to the white manager on all matters, as he was the real line manager, not the black manager.
- He had the overall control of the project, including finance, and had the final say in the project outcome.
- He took the leading role in reporting to the steering committee and decided how, when and which members of the committee were to be involved or consulted and for what purpose.

Although the above agenda was not formalised explicitly, the manner in which the white manager carried out his management responsibilities made it quite apparent to the black manager and the project worker. The black manager and the project worker also realised that the white manager's agenda was not only undermining their roles in the project, but it was also restricting their valuable contributions to the project as well. In addition, they were fully aware of the fact that the white manager's agenda would be against the interest of the black and minority ethnic communities, if the project process and outcome were toned down to avoid upsetting the white audiences.

In order to counteract the white manager's agenda, the black manager and the project worker began to establish an alternative management agenda. This focused on:

- ensuring that the project gained the confidence of black and minority ethnic communities
- adopting methods and approaches in the project processes and outcomes which could minimise the credibility of the project to the black constituency
- using the project as an aid to advocate for better services to black and minority ethnic families and influence policy makers and service providers
- involving as many black and minority ethnic professionals and groups as possible within the project work
- developing strategies for co-working with white professionals and managers and forming an alliance with them with a view to strengthening the work of the project.

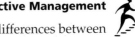

forward the following pointers illustrating the differences between the white and black accountability in this context.

- For the white manager, the project was accountable primarily to the funding agency and then to the white audience. For the black manager and the project worker, the project was mainly accountable to the black and minority ethnic professionals, groups and communities.
- Because the black manager and the project worker developed their management agenda jointly, they established a joint ownership of management issues, making them accountable to each other in pursuing their joint agenda. The white manager did not feel that he was accountable to his black colleagues, although he was inclined to be accountable to the funding authority. Furthermore, his perception of 'controlling' the project, and hence the black manager and the project worker too, meant that the two black members of the project were accountable to him.
- While the white manager juxtaposed accountability in the power structure and power relationships, the black duo placed theirs in the hands of the powerless.

Ahmed concluded with a number of issues which need to be addressed if black and minority ethnic managers are to maintain their cultural pride and professional credibility whilst carrying out their roles.

- Black managers should not be hindered but actively enabled to make positive use of their community experiences (accountability being one of them).
- Accountability to the community and to their organisation should not be seen as conflicting interests and they should not come under pressure to be 'loyal' to the organisations first and to be 'accountable' to the communities last.
- It is in the interest of the organisation to encourage its black managers to promote their management accountability and make contributions to enhancing the accountability of the institutions.
- Organisations should recognise that their black managers cannot and should not be expected to behave as surrogate traditional white managers.
- Services need to appreciate that compartmentalising of management and caring duties and responsibilities should be seen as undesirable and that without actively implementing their advocacy roles, black managers cannot make the services 'user

The multiracial team: the challenges ahead

sensitive' to meet the needs of the 'clients'. Nor can they advocate for necessary changes in their agencies, without which the services cannot achieve their caring objectives and welfare goals.

- The role of advocacy should be one of the vital pivots of management and should be a management criterion for all, instead of the tendency to label managers (especially those from minority ethnic groups) who advocate for their service users as trouble-makers.

References

Acheson D 1998 Independent inquiry into inequalities in health. Stationery Office, London

Ahmed B 1980 Community social work: sharing the experience of ethnic groups. Social Work Today, 14 July, p 13

Ahmed B 1992 Dictionary of black managers in white organisations. Race Equality Unit, National Institute of Social Work, London

Beishon S, Virdee S, Hagell A 1995 Nursing in a multiethnic NHS. Policy Studies Institute, London

Commission for Racial Equality 1983 Ethnic minority hospital staff. CRE, London

Cox T 1991 Managing the multi-cultural organisation. Journal of the Academy of Management Executives 5(2): 34–37

Department of Health 1992 The health of the nation. HMSO, London

Department of Health 2000 Summit on the recruitment and retention of black and ethnic minority staff in the NHS, October 25. Department of Health, London

European Commission 1999 Report from the Commission on the implementation of European Year Against Racism. European Community, The Hague, The Netherlands

Kanter R M 1977 Men and women of the corporation. Basic Books, New York

King's Fund 1990 Racial equality in the nursing professions. Occasional Paper No. 6. King's Fund, London

Lee-Cunin M 1989 Daughters of Seacole: a study of black nurses in West Yorkshire. West Yorkshire Low Pay Unit, Batley

McEnrue M P 1993 Managing diversity: Los Angeles before and after the riots. Organisational Dynamics 21(3): 18–29

Macpherson W (Chair) 1999 The Stephen Lawrence inquiry. Stationery Office, London

OPCS 1993 1991 Census: ethnic group and country of birth. Great Britain, Volume 2. HMSO, London

Royal College of Physicians 1993 Access to health care for people from black and ethnic minorities. Royal College of Physicians, London

Smage C 1995 Health, race and ethnicity: making sense of the evidence. King's Fund, London

Application 11:1
Carol Baxter, Peter Toon

Nurses, doctors and the meaning of holism: interprofessionalism and values in primary care

INTRODUCTION

There has been a historical tradition of mutual dependence amongst the workforce in the NHS. Current systems of service delivery are requiring even closer collaboration and joint working between the different health and care professionals and disciplines. The move towards interprofessionalism, a key factor in the government's modernisation agenda for the NHS (Health Secretary 1996), is based upon the view that all participants bring equally valid knowledge and expertise from their professional and personal experience and that a 'diverse group can arrive at a place no individual and no like-minded group would have reached' (Davis 2000).

What is often not explored, however, are the questions and challenges arising from differences in values amongst professional groups which motivate their practice and influence their attitudes and beliefs about what is best for patients. Our fundamental values have an enormous influence on the way we approach our work of which we are not always aware. Such an understanding on the part of individual professionals is, however, particularly important in the primary care context where the newly formed primary care trusts are required to promote individual and organisational commitment to quality, equity, corporate behaviour and public accountability. The extent to which this will be affected by professional culture clashes is yet to be seen.

Research which has helped to develop our understanding in this area was carried out by the National Primary Care Research and Development Centre (Williams et al 1997). Focusing on the introduction of the internal market in the early 1990s, the study set out to identify core values in nursing, how these differed from those of medicine and which distinct aspects of care may be lost or gained as primary care nurses substitute for general practitioners. The underlying hypothesis was that the rapid changes in the roles of health care professionals created problems of insecurity and loss of identity for many and that this sometimes increased defensiveness and impaired effective collaboration. The main methods of data collection were via a systematic detailed literature review of nursing, medicine, sociology and health service research. This was backed up by in-depth interviews with 15 respondents considered to be key commentators in both nursing and medicine.

One of the major findings of this study was the differing perspectives on holism held by the two professional groups, detailed in the extract presented in Box 11.1.1.

> **Box 11.1.1** Differing perspectives on holism of doctors and nurses (from Williams et al 1997)
>
> Nurses have taken over a number of roles which GPs formerly held. This is regretted by many GPs, in part because it challenges their notion of 'holistic' care since they are no longer the sole provider of all aspects of primary health care to each patient. Thus there is a sense in which GPs experience a loss as work moves to practice nurses. Further, this is expressed as not merely a loss to GPs, but also to patients. One GP commented that 'disease is about dealing with families', and from her point of view, nursing's assumption of health promotion and prevention in some areas was cutting into a GP's relationship with the holistic care of the family. This suggestion broadly accords with contributors to the literature (including Richardson & Maynard 1995 and Garbett 1996). There is a suggestion of a hint of concern for the potential loss to patients should a holistic generalist perspective be compromised by work undertaken by nurses.
>
> Of course, nurses also use the word holistic to describe the care they give (May 1991, 1992). When pressed to distinguish how her care might differ from the care of a doctor a practice nurse who was interviewed for the study suggested:
>
> > *I think they do deal with caring. I think the whole holistic approach of medicine is caring, but I feel they care more from a treatment point of view. They care enough to listen to the symptoms and get them (patients) the best possible treatment ... nursing care comes more from the emotional side ... There*

Box 11.1.1   Cont'd

*are different types of care. And their (doctors') care is in getting
the treatment, the diagnosis … where nursing care is more from
the social point of view and more on a level as well. I do
think lots of patients see doctors as being up on a pedestal.*
(Interview 11)

The study suggests that there are differences between the meanings
attributed by doctors and nurses to the connections between holism,
relationships and care. GPs' care is holistic in terms of dealing with all
aspects of a person's health, shaped by their generalist perspective.
In the words of one GP in the study:

*Our work is defined by relationships … and if you say (referring
to a patient) well actually she's got this disease and she should
go to that clinic (run by a practice nurse) then that cuts our
whole approach which is about relationships and people and it's
about working with disease.* (Interview 1)

In contrast, nurses see no conflict with specialism vs holism since care
is shaped by knowing the individual as a whole person and mutual
sharing of experiences. Nursing the whole person is a fairly common
expression in nursing literature pertaining to nurse–patient
relationships (Fagermoen 1997, Prior 1996, Spooner 1995) and
holism, in this way, is part of the discourse of nursing (Owen &
Holmes 1993).

A key point is that if GPs are holistic in terms of dealing with the
overall medical status of patients, then they need to be generalist in
their skills. If nurses are holistic in terms of dealing with patients'
emotional and social needs it could be argued that they do not need
to be generalist, but that they can take account of emotional and
social needs in relation to particular conditions or diseases. In short,
they act as specialists in relation to the condition. It is interesting to
note that within nursing discourse, very little discussion of holism in
relation to generalism appears in the literature, whereas links are
made between holism and specialism (Ward-Miller 1996, Whitehead
1996, Love 1995, Choi 1995).

Thus both GPs and nurses are feeling some sense of loss during
this period of change, and both are finding they cannot exploit
holism, and other hard-to-define aspects of care, as much as
they would like. As one of the respondents pointed out,
'despite the fact that nurses are trained in holism, the concept
is totally unmarketable in the current climate'. A possible
explanation of this is the current tendency to value what is
easily measurable (by quantitative performance indicators)
rather than to measure hard-to-define but valuable concepts, such
as 'holistic' care.

Nurses, doctors and the meaning of holism

DISCUSSION

The differences in power, education, pay, status, class and gender between doctors and nurses are well recognised and documented. In commenting on the power relationships between the two professional groups, Davis (2000) states:

> Traditionally the profession of medicine emphasised expertise, autonomy and responsibility more than interdependence, deliberation and dialogue. Nursing on the other hand emphasises hierarchy and bureaucracy even if these have diminished along with deference to doctors; nurses still work around others.

It is the differences in unspoken assumptions, however, which can often lead to the greatest confusion and can impact most profoundly on standards of patient care. General practice, for example, places great value on the continuity of care of patients by individual practitioners, whilst nurse managers tend to see nurses much more as interchangeable and the provision of continuity of service as a key value. When a district nurse or health visitor attached to a practice is moved by her manager to another position for reasons which (in terms of maintaining an equitable service) seem perfectly rational to a nurse manager, it may seem capricious to a general practitioner who has just got to know her and who feels 'she has just got to know the patients'.

PROFESSIONAL DEVELOPMENT AND SUPPORT

If the thinking behind the actions was made clear from the outset, then dialogue to avert unnecessary frustration and damage to relationships could have been facilitated. It is hard to look at the ground under your feet and to be explicit about your values. This skill rarely occurs naturally but can be cultivated. Increasingly, professional development and support are being recognised for their important role in addressing interprofessional differences and enhancing collaborative working.

In the case of nurses and doctors, such developments are based on the premise that traditionally, the approach to training offered little chance for them to meet before they arrive on the wards: the tendency is for them to be trained and socialised mainly within their own discipline. Thus, many of the problems arise at an early stage. In addition to the setting, there are also significant differences in the underlying rationale. Nursing has a tradition of formal, centrally accredited courses and of strictly limiting practice to areas of proven competence. Medicine, in contrast, leaves the individual doctor both to determine his or her own learning needs and to define the limits of competence.

In the UK these two traditions are moving closer together, as self-directed learning through methods such as clinical supervision,

The diverse team – making it work

mentoring and reflective journals become more popular in nursing, whilst the failure of autonomous individual self-regulation in medical practice in a number of well-publicised cases has led to calls for revalidation and appraisal systems.

The recognition of the need for competent interprofessional working is now a key aspect of the reforms in health professional education. Attention is being paid to this not only through initiatives in the curricula of uniprofessional courses but also in the development of programmes of joint or shared learning (Barr & Shaw 1995). Development in interprofessional competencies or capabilities in essence addresses the specialist knowledge, values and skills professionals require to undertake effective joint working in the service of users.

Boxes 11.1.2 and 11.1.3 summarise some of the barriers to and success factors for effective professional collaboration.

CONCLUSION

The field of primary care is indeed a very rich testing ground for what will become increasingly important not only in hospitals but also across traditional boundaries of health and social care. Gregson et al (1991) remind us of the value of focusing on the concept of collaboration in a meaningful way; the greater the understanding gained, the greater the potential for improved joint working and raised standards of care. They refer to the importance of clarifying differing perceptions, values, expectations, assumptions, behaviours and structures which shape the nature of collaboration in and across health and social care settings.

Box 11.1.2 Success factors for working in an interdisciplinary team (from Weinstein 1998)

Common understanding of goals and objectives
Clear jargon-free communication
Effective leadership
Regular interaction between members
Equal participation by and valuing of all members
Meaningful and challenging tasks for all participants
Joint evaluation and joint planning
Clear decision-making processes
Small enough numbers of people to facilitate thorough and regular communication
Open acknowledgement of power issues related to hierarchy, status, race, gender and other structural differences
Recognition of the unique contribution of each member of the team

---

Nurses, doctors and the meaning of holism

The diverse team – making it work

> **Box 11.1.3** Barriers to interdisciplinary functioning (from Weinstein 1998)
>
> Lack of shared aims and goals
> Different language/jargon
> Conflicting values/ethics/attitudes
> Different cultures
> Status differences – minority dominate
> Race and gender issues – lack of involvement and participation by key members
> Lack of knowledge about each other's roles
> Lack of clarity about tasks and responsibility
> Power struggles
> Unexpressed conflict leading to poor communication and distrust
> Inability/unwillingness to share
> Lack of knowledge about group/organisational dynamics
> Lack of self-awareness
> Rigid and narrow view of remit
> Lack of clarity about interagency procedures and decision-making processes
> Size of team too large for successful interaction

Discussion questions

As a nurse manager with responsibility for professional development what strategies would you recommend for training and support of nurses and doctros to work more effectively together? Would you support:

- Common foundation year as a basis for further uniprofessional training?
- More joint training and shared learning throughout qualifying training?
- Focusing more on job development and training at the postqualifying stage?

How would you justify your preferences?

References

Barr H, Shaw I 1995 Shared learning: selected examples from the literature. CAIPE, London

Choi M 1995 The menopausal transition: change, loss and adaptation. Holistic Nursing Practice 9(3):53–62

Davis C 2000 Vive la difference: that's what will make collaboration work. Nursing Times 96(15):27

Fagermoen M 1997 Professional identity: values embedded in meaningful nursing practices. Journal of Advanced Nursing 25:434–441

Garbett R 1996 The growth of nurse-led care. Nursing Times 92(1):29

Gregson B, Cartilidge A, Bond J 1991 Interprofessional collaboration in primary care organisations. Occasional paper 52. Royal College of General Practitioners, London

Health Secretary 1996 The new NHS: modern, dependable. HMSO, London

Love C 1995 Orthopaedic nursing: a study of its specialist status. Nursing Standard 9 (44):36–40

May C 1991 Nursing work, nurses' knowledge and the subjectification of the patient. Sociology of Health and Illness 14(4):472–487

May C 1992 Affective neutrality and involvement in nurse–patient relationships: perceptions of appropriate behaviour among nurses in acute medical and surgical wards. Journal of Advanced Nursing 16:552–558

Owen M, Holmes C 1993 Holism in the discourse of nursing. Journal of Advanced Nursing 18:1688–1695

Prior I 1996 Caring for patients from ethnic minority groups. British Journal of Theatre Nursing 6(3):28–30

Richardson G, Maynard A 1995 Fewer doctors? More nurses? A review of the knowledge base of doctor–nurse substitution. Discussion paper 135. Centre for Development of Interprofessional Education, University of York

Spooner A 1995 A personal perspective: the psychological needs of spine injured patients. Professional Nurse 10(6):359–362

Ward-Miller S 1996 The psychiatric clinical specialist in the home-care setting. Nursing Clinics of North America 31(3):519–525

Weinstein J 1998 The professions and their inter-relationships. In: Thompson J, Mathias P (eds) Standards and learning disability. Baillière Tindall, London

Whitehead C 1996 The specialist nurse in HIV/AIDs medicine. Postgraduate Medical Journal 72(846):211–213

Williams A, Robins T, Sibbald B 1997 Cultural differences between medicine and nursing: implications for primary care. National Primary Care Research and Development Centre, Manchester University

Nurses, doctors and the meaning of holism

Application 11:2
Bob Sapey

Collaborating for effectiveness: a disability project

The diverse team – making it work

In 1986 the Audit Commission criticised the funding of residential and nursing homes in the independent sector, through Income Support payments from the Department of Social Security, as offering a 'perverse incentive' to local authorities not to provide community care which would have to be paid for out of their social service departments' budgets. Subsequently, the Griffiths Report *Agenda for action*, the government White Paper *Caring for people* and the National Health Service and Community Care Act 1990 all aimed to remove this incentive and to promote collaboration between health, housing and social service authorities.

However, in 1998 the Audit Commission once again reported and this time they described the community care budgetary arrangements that had been constructed as having created a 'Berlin wall' between health and social service agencies. While it is clear that these barriers are the result of government decisions and action, it remains the responsibility of welfare professionals who are working directly with disabled people to ensure that services are effective and this often means having to overcome the structural barriers that have been created by politicians and accountants.

In this chapter I shall look at one attempt at collaboration which took place in the 1980s in order to see what can be learnt for practising in the current structures.

A SCHEDULED MEETING OF PEOPLE

Community rehabilitation teams were formed in the early 1980s following the successful collaboration between a range of health and social work professionals who were working with a young man who had severe head injuries. The need to offer a community-based rehabilitation programme for this man arose in part because of the Falklands War, which had led to many rehabilitation centres being full, and in part to the negative attitude of other centres which simply wanted to institutionalise him. On analysing the services available in the rehabilitation centres, it was clear that they were no different to those available in the community but they were extremely well coordinated. The result of this individual programme was comparatively successful but it also demonstrated the ability of people to work together.

These teams were not teams in the usual organisational sense of being sited in one place and employed within a single agency. Rather, they were made up of doctors, nurses, social workers, occupational therapists, physiotherapists, speech therapists, psychologists, housing officers, disablement resettlement officers and home helps on an ad hoc basis according to the needs of individual disabled people. It was in reality a scheduled meeting of people, who were working in hospitals and the community, at which they liaised and cooperated in their treatment and care of an individual. What this achieved was the ability to offer a programme of rehabilitation, rather than just a range of specialist services. At its simplest and yet most effective level, what the team did was to ensure that services were started as they became necessary and to continue treatment to fill in gaps in a programme. So, for example, if the DRO was arranging a work placement which could not start immediately, the OT might continue her treatment beyond what she would have done if she had been working in isolation, in order to ensure the individual did not have to spend time waiting without any therapy. This type of collaboration proved very successful for a number of people and meant that the community services of a relatively remote part of the country were able to rival those of many specialised rehabilitation centres. Indeed, if one considers the tendency of such centres to make the negative recommendation of permanent nursing home care, this community service was much better.

PRACTITIONERS RATHER THAN MANAGERS

A key feature of these teams was that they were made up of practitioners rather than managers. The team was concerned with the negotiation of a service for an individual and in that sense it was appropriate that it should be the practitioners involved with their care and treatment who should be meeting. While resources might be controlled elsewhere, in practice it was found that a practitioner holding the team recommendation was in a very good position to negotiate the use of those resources. Had the teams been made up of managers, there would have been the danger of them letting

Collaborating for effectiveness

their resource concerns affect the professional recommendations and indeed, it may have been too remote from the disabled person to be of any value. Of course, many professionals had some control over resources and at the very least they had control over themselves as a resource, but this did not prevent them from acting in the interests of their patient or client.

However, what was noticeable was the impact on these teams of the restructuring and reorganisation of both health and social services. As health trusts began to work to prescribed contracts with GPs and the district health authority, it became more difficult for individual practitioners to determine the use of their own time or to provide help from the resources under their management. Their contracts were prepared too far in advance to be able to predict the needs of individuals and as a result the services became rigid. Similarly, in the social services, when the purchaser–provider splits were brought in, there developed a lengthy negotiation over each individual request for a service. Services that had been available on the basis of professional recommendation became rationed, not because they were unavailable but because they had to be accounted for by proceduralised criteria. In both authorities the culture was changing from one of collaboration to one of budget protectionism – saying 'no' rather than 'yes'. The teams were also susceptible to incorporation within the mainstream bureaucracies of the health and social services authorities. While they worked effectively as an ad hoc structure, once management had expectations of the teams as part of the formal liaison between their agencies, this inevitably led to them being dominated by non-practitioners and they tended to take on a self-sustaining life of their own. As with any other bureaucratic organisation, this tendency often runs counter to effective action.

The final issue was that of client/patient participation. The issue of participation is important to disabled people and while some individuals working in the welfare sector take this seriously, others fail to recognise its value. From my own observations, what I saw was an initial attempt to include disabled people but as the teams became more formal, this became less desirable. The difficulty was that as participation became more important to disabled people, so it became more difficult in the very structures that sought to make services more effective. Again, this is very clear in the literature on participation; if people are to be involved then the structure of meetings needs to enable it. Participation is not something that can be done by simply inviting a relatively powerless individual to join in an established group of powerful professionals. This is disempowering and leads to a very effective exclusion of the individual. What is needed is for those involved to understand the impact of their welfare professionalism on patients/clients and to provide support and structures that enable inclusion within the decision-making process.

LESSONS LEARNT

There are lessons to be learnt from this. First and foremost is that effectiveness appears to be achieved when collaboration is informal and specifically aimed at improving the services for a particular individual. While it is tempting to formalise the arrangements that worked well for one person and apply them to others, this may not be the best approach. However, when the same small group of individuals are involved with a number of people there are obvious advantages to developing some structures that are more efficient than many separate meetings. This is a matter of managing the right balance of formalisation while not incorporating the structure as a permanent part of the bureaucracy. It also means accepting that collaborative arrangements may need to be time limited if they are to give way to the next round of collaboration.

This type of structural arrangement is called networking and observations of successful technological industries throughout the world show this to be a core feature of their organisation. Networks are formed because they support collaborative strategies but once these have been achieved, they need to be dissolved in order to make space for the next strategic network.

A further issue concerns the rigidity of the funding arrangements within which most welfare professions now work. Clearly it is not practical or possible to ignore these structures, no matter how damaging they are, but there are positive and negative ways of working within them. The first obstacle to overcome is the temptation to follow the example of senior managers and always refuse a service or seek to have it paid for by another agency. It is much better to say 'yes' and then discuss funding responsibilities rather than to say 'no' and then fight. Collaboration, like any other relationship, involves give and take. If both parties set out to take, the relationship soon falls apart. Collaboration is a difficult and time-consuming task but if the effectiveness of therapy and care is dependent upon it, then it is counterproductive not to do so enthusiastically. Collaboration needs to be based on mutual trust rather than suspicion and while the budgetary structures of health and social services may promote the latter, it remains a duty of welfare workers to foster the former in their professional relationships.

Finally, there is little point in establishing good collaborative arrangements that exclude the most significant person – the recipient of the services. Strategies need to be worked out to ensure participation. This may be through an ambassadorial approach where one worker acts as go-between or it may mean all parties concerned meeting together, including the patient/client. Participation will meet resistance from some professionals but this should be challenged. There are virtually no circumstances where it is in the interests of a disabled person to be excluded from the decisions being made by health and welfare agencies; rather, it is often justified in this way in order to make life more comfortable for the welfare professionals. Again, this is a case of a professional responsibility to include, rather than exclude disabled people from their own lives.

Application 11:3
Lai Fong Chiu

Extending the team outwards: building partnerships and teamwork with communities

INTRODUCTION

The notion of partnership has been highlighted as the crucial underpinning of the new initiatives in the NHS. Patient access to services and their empowerment are also major modernisation challenges, thus the notion of partnership must include patients as partners in service design implementation, monitoring and delivery. This is particularly important in primary care trusts, where teamwork skills among staff are crucial to the capacity for building successful partnerships within and between general practices and with users. It is important for general practices to facilitate a teamwork culture and establish provision for systematic learning of teamwork skills, not only to enhance the capacity of their staff but also to facilitate the building of partnerships with local communities as engines by which quality services may be developed and delivered.

This chapter presents the author's practical experience in facilitating the extension of practice teams to include lay members of the communities in a health promotion initiative that addresses the inequality of access of minority ethnic women to the cervical screening service using the community health educator's model (Chiu 1993, 1998, Chiu et al 1993).

THE COMMUNITY HEALTH EDUCATOR'S MODEL

The community health educator model was initially developed from an action research project entitled *Communicating breast screening messages to minority women* (Chiu 1993). The major thrust of the model is the use of bilingual women volunteers from different minority ethnic communities to take on the role of health educators and promoters within their own communities. These volunteers were subjected to an intensive period of training which included knowledge in breast health and cancer, skills in adult education, one-to-one and group work, project organisation and evaluation. As community health educators (CHEs), they were then paid to carry out health education and promotion work with women from their communities on a sessional basis.

The model was further refined in the primary care setting through another action research project entitled *Woman-to-woman: promoting cervical screening among minority ethnic women in primary care* (Chiu 1998). It used a partnership approach to promote cervical screening involving six general practices in the South Yorkshire area. Six minority ethnic communities, Pakistani (Mirpuri), Bengali (Sylheti), Chinese (Cantonese), African-Caribbean (English), Yemeni (Arabic), were targeted. The smear takers of the participating practices and the bilingual women formed a professional and lay team to tackle low attendance rates of smear tests and to promote women's health. Within a 6-month period, six CHEs had made visits to women in their communities to carry out prescreening health education. They also made practice link visits and spent time in supporting women in accessing screening and other services in primary care.

The balance of activities varied widely among different language groups due to the varying needs of the women in the communities. For example, due to the high language support needs in clinical situations, the Chinese (Cantonese) CHE spent a great deal of time in supporting women during smear testing or accessing other services, while the African-Caribbean CHE spent more time in group or one-to-one health education and promotion activities in her community. CHEs also worked with the enlisted practices focusing on carrying out health education with non-attenders. Did Not Attend (DNA) lists were provided by two general practices and a 66% improvement in uptake of cervical screening following CHEs' visits was found in these practices (Chiu 1998).

PRACTICE AND COMMUNITY PARTNERSHIP CONFIGURATION

Although the ideal situation for putting together the partnership was to pair up each CHE with a smear taker in a practice with substantial numbers of the minority population to which the CHE belonged, it was not always possible to have such a symmetrical relationship between community groups and general practices. The

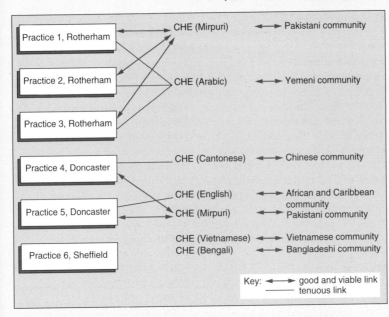

Figure 11.3.1. The actual configuration of primary care partnerships

actual configuration of the relationships between CHEs who represented the six language groups involved is illustrated in Figure 11.3.1.

Although the configuration seemed complex, the matrix arrangement of teamwork, in which the one-to-one partnerships formed on the local practice level were regrouped as partnerships between CHEs and smear takers across localities on another level, has made it possible to deal with great diversity. For instance, because the CHEs were working as a team, some of the enlisted practices were able to draw on their support to serve the smaller scattered local communities such as the Cantonese, Yemeni and Vietnamese.

KEY COMPONENTS IN BUILDING THE TEAM OUTWARDS

On reflection, the following were crucial components in building such teams with the communities:

- self-assessment
- mutual respect
- goal setting
- commitment to learning cycles
- conflict resolution
- inclusive evaluation.

Extending the team outwards

Self-assessment

The project provided opportunities for both the smear takers from the enlisted practices and women from the targeted communities to assess their situations and express their concerns regarding the issue of promoting cervical screening among women from minority ethnic communities. These discussions were facilitated in focus groups in which smear takers and minority ethnic women of each community could identify their concerns and find solutions to resolve these concerns. Both professional and lay perceptions of the issue were then presented back to each group. Taking a problem focus (cervical screening) to self-assessment allowed both professionals and communities to relate to a concrete issue. With the emergence of different perspectives, both professional and communities were able to reorientate themselves towards a common goal, i.e. collectively formulating a health promotion strategy for cervical screening.

Mutual respect

When the first-time smear takers and communities (represented here by the bilingual CHEs) came together to implement the health promotion strategy, it was not surprising that there were suspicions, stereotyping and prejudices on both sides. Critical learning workshops were introduced in which the participants' preconceptions and attitudes were challenged. These workshops consisted of participants learning about the impacts of discriminatory practices, critically reviewing their own cultural knowledge and practices vis-à-vis minority communities in the contemporary British context and becoming aware of the language and communication of discrimination as well as the potential contribution of the bilingual members of the communities in clinical interactions. These critical workshops had the effect of raising professional participants' awareness of the inequality that they might help to perpetuate and of the unequal power relationships that underpinned the interactions between professionals and lay members of the communities. This ultimately led to the establishment of mutual respect between professionals and communities.

Goal setting

Once mutual respect had been established, the smear takers and the CHEs were able to give meaning to their involvement in the project and were able to envision the ultimate goals that they wished to achieve. Those professionals who were able to form links directly with a locally residing CHE quickly set themselves goals that were appropriate to their local situation. For example, the practice in Rotherham and the local Pakistani (Mirpuri) CHE decided to tackle the DNA list first. Since there was no ethnic monitoring in place, the CHE assisted in the identification of Pakistani women who had failed to attend the smear test. Their ultimate goal was to improve the uptake among non-attenders. Other CHE/smear taker partnerships established different goals, e.g. the setting up of women's health promotion clinics based in their practices.

Commitment to learning cycles

Within the period of implementation of the health promotion strategy, there were regular research subgroup meetings in which participants could bring forth any problems or issues arising from their work. There was a climate of open communication and learning and innovative ways of solving problems were encouraged. For example, in supporting women for their smear tests, a number of the CHEs found that they were continually treated by other professionals (smear takers in family clinics or other non-enlisted practices) as uninformed 'relatives' of service users instead of equal partners in delivering a quality smear test service. This made it difficult for the CHEs to facilitate dialogue between the smear takers and service users. The problem was discussed in one of the subgroup meetings and a collective solution was found. The subgroup decided to issue a blanket official communication to all practices and family planning clinics across the districts and an in-service training workshop on assertion and advocacy was conducted. The result has been a significant improvement of the working relationships between CHEs and other health professionals across the districts. This demonstrated the importance of gaining everyone's commitment to the principle of learning cycles. Not only is this necessary for effective solution of problems, but this participative approach to problem solving helps to cement relationships and improve mutual respect in the partnerships.

Conflict resolution

In partnership working between professionals and lay members of the communities, conflict is unavoidable. Skills in handling conflicts are important for the growth and development of the partnership. Unresolved conflicts may have the potential to damage the project and not only to wreck relationships on which the success of the project depends, but also to bring emotional harm to people involved. One of the examples of conflict that we successfully resolved was the question of payments to CHEs. The smear takers were surprised and upset when they inadvertently found out that the hourly rate of pay of the CHEs was similar to their own. Their immediate reaction was that they felt that their professional knowledge and expertise were not valued. However, the smear takers were placated when it was explained that the CHEs, rate of

Extending the team outwards

pay reflected their own special skills and the temporary nature of their employment.

Inclusive evaluation

The development of evaluation methods in partnership working and team building needs to move away from focusing only on the objective assessment of goals attainment to a more sophisticated and complex approach that accounts for the multiple realities, interests and values of team members and partners. It is also important to recognise that outcomes of team working depend heavily upon relationship building and team processes. Therefore, while an agreed approach to formulating success criteria remains central to team-work evaluation, the opportunities for process-oriented evaluation should not be overlooked. The combination of process and outcome evaluation underpinned by multiple perspectives could give us insights for future improvement. In the Woman-to-Woman project, although the focus group method was the main vehicle for evaluation, individual team members were allowed opportunities to reflect on team processes with a facilitator when each milestone of the project had been reached.

CONCLUSION

Although teamwork is not a new concept, the recent rallying cry for partnership within the NHS modernisation movement has made it more urgent for us to integrate it into our ways of working. Based upon my experience with the Woman-to-Woman project, this chapter has offered some insights for those who wish to extend their partnerships outwards to a diverse community. The key components of developing professional and lay partnership discussed here are neither exhaustive nor in themselves mutually exclusive. The practice of team working with communities requires imagination, innovation and courage. I hope this example will encourage other practitioners to consider applying this approach in working with the community.

References

Chiu L F (ed) 1993 Communicating breast screening messages to minority women: a conference report. Leeds Health Promotion Service, Leeds

Chiu L F 1998 Woman-To-woman: promoting cervical screening among minority ethnic women in primary care, a participatory action research project (1995–1997). A research report. Department of Health Promotion, Rotherham Health Authority, Rotherham

Chiu L F, Knight D, Williams S 1993 Breast screening training pack for minority women. Leeds Health Promotion Service, Leeds

The diverse team – making it work

Section **Six**

DIVERSITY AND SERVICE QUALITY

Chapter **Twelve**

Clinical governance

Salman Rawaf, Kelly Powell

OVERVIEW

The purpose of this chapter is to introduce the reader to the concept of clinical governance and to emphasise the part that managing diversity has to play in making clinical governance successful. It begins by defining clinical governance and describing the background that resulted in the need for the clinical governance system. It follows with a description of the tools available to set, monitor and evaluate standards of care and describes the new statutory requirements of the various NHS bodies. The chapter concludes that managers can implement diversity theory in order to harness the differences between both individuals and groups in order to best serve the organisation and in doing so, improve the quality of care that patients receive.

INTRODUCTION

The White Paper *The new NHS: modern, dependable* stated the government's concern with inconsistent, poor-quality clinical care and for the first time gave all health organisations in the NHS a statutory duty to seek quality improvement through a defined system of 'clinical governance'. This is a very important step since for the first time it places on health care managers a statutory responsibility for quality of clinical care on an equal footing with the preexisting duty of financial responsibility.

DEFINITION

Clinical governance is:

> a system through which all of the organisations in the National Health Service are accountable for continuously improving the quality of their clinical services and ensuring high standards of patient care by creating a facilitative environment in which excellence will flourish. (Chief Medical Officer 1999)

- It is basically a framework for the improvement of patient care through commitment to high standards, reflective practice, risk management and personal and team development.
- It is about providing the best possible clinical care for patients, identifying and avoiding areas of high risk in patient care and making the most effective use of available resources.
- It is about the individual clinical responsibilities of doctors, nurses and other health care staff and the collective responsibility of the team, service or organisation and the balance between them.
- It aims to put high-quality care at the heart of all decisions made, at whatever level, within the NHS.

The easiest way to think about how we all fit into the clinical governance model is to consider duties at each level within the organisation: the individual, the department or directorate and then the organisation itself.

Management can contribute greatly to the success of clinical governance by harnessing the very different subcultures that work within the NHS and realising that different attitudes and approaches can be good for the organisation. They need to ensure that these different groups do not feel threatened by differences of approach or opinion and are willing and able to work together.

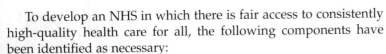
To develop an NHS in which there is fair access to consistently high-quality health care for all, the following components have been identified as necessary:

- clear national standards
- mechanisms for ensuring local delivery of these standards
- mechanisms for monitoring the delivery of these standards.

Standards will be set at a national level with the development of National Service Frameworks (NSFs), to cover whole service areas such as, for example, mental health and coronary heart disease, and the National Institute for Clinical Excellence (NICE) to cover individual treatments, for example new drugs. It will obviously take time to envelop all the important areas of health care so in many clinical areas, local standards will be set in the intervening period. These local standards must be shown to be based on the best available evidence.

Mechanisms to ensure local delivery of these clinical standards are the responsibility of the local trusts and the health authority (for public health and primary care groups).

Monitoring of standards will be undertaken both locally (by the trusts, the health authority and primary care groups) and nationally (by the Commission for Health Improvement and the National Survey of Patient and User Experiences).

RATIONALE

The White Paper *The new NHS: modern, dependable* stated the government's concern with inconsistent, poor-quality clinical care. The 1990 NHS reforms put the emphasis on finance and stimulated quantity – rather than quality-driven competition.

This was highlighted by a number of well-publicised serious failures in clinical care, like the Bristol paediatric cardiothoracic deaths and failures in breast and cervical cancer screening, and made worse by obvious but hard-to-explain variations in standards and clinical care and by major inquiries into service failures. In order to regain public confidence and trust, it was necessary to emphasise the importance of clinical quality, hence the inception of clinical governance. It is important to realise that clinical governance does not imply entirely new activity, since much of the work needed to ensure best possible care is already taking place. However, a more systematic approach is needed to ensure good practice is recognised and shared and bad practice is changed.

Clinical governance

Six Steps to **Effective Management**

In order to best effect good patient outcome, a sea change in attitudes must be accomplished. Changing the workplace behaviour of individual practitioners will require a variety of interventions if it is to be successful. A complex process has to be planned to include the early stages of training and should include altering the structure in which they train and work (see Box 12.1).

THE RELATIONSHIP BETWEEN CLINICAL GOVERNANCE AND MANAGING DIVERSITY

Managing diversity is about being aware of the potential of individuals' differences to benefit the organisation and actively encouraging the development of these differences. It builds on the legal framework of equal opportunities but does not restrict itself to the area set out by law. By valuing differences it allows individuals to develop their full potential, whatever their background, culture, sex, political affiliation or age, and ensures that they feel they are playing an important part in the organisation's business. Within the NHS, there are many individuals who 'do their own thing'. Managers can embrace this individuality if it is based on the best evidence available.

The professional groups that work in the NHS (managerial and clinical) tend to have very different backgrounds and training and very different philosophical approaches to patient care. Historically, this has often resulted in politicking and conflict. This diversity should be viewed in a more positive way by both managers and the groups themselves and it is the role of the manager to ensure that this happens.

NECESSARY TOOLS

There are a number of tools available that can be utilised in the three areas of setting (identifying), applying and monitoring standards. To operate an effective and smooth-running clinical governance system, these components must be interlinked and work interdependently. The role of management is to ensure system maintenance ('oiling the system'), clear lines of accountability, transparency of reporting and action to implement change, as well as determining which diverse attitudes and practices will benefit patient care. The main tools are described below.

Clinical audit

This is a very important tool for clinical governance but audit should not become the goal itself. Instead, it should be used to encourage clinicians to work to preset standards and frequently

Clinical governance

review the quality of care they provide, making improvements where necessary. Many attempts at audit in the past have not gone beyond the setting standards and measuring performance stage. It is imperative that standards and performance are then compared and acted on in an appropriate manner. For this to become user friendly, trusts and PCGs will need to develop systems to collect high-quality, useful information routinely and a blaming culture must be avoided. To make audit appropriate to diversity, we need to ensure that audits look at access, utilisation and outcomes in different groups, by age, sex, ethnicity, disability and so on.

Research and development

This forms the basis for evidence-based medicine. The NHS Research and Development Strategy was launched in 1991 to develop a knowledge-based NHS where decisions (clinical, policy and managerial) would have a sound base. This will continue to have a pivotal role in collecting new evidence, with support from the Horizon Scanning Centre and the National Prescribing Centre in identifying new and existing interventions. Consumer involvement in research is becoming more commonplace, with the use of questionnaire surveys and focus groups, and this should be encouraged in the name of diversity.

Evidence-based medicine

The White Papers make it clear that effective, integrated health care must be grounded, where possible, on an evidence base and the NICE has been set up to spearhead best practice throughout the NHS. However, much work has already been done by the Cochrane Collaboration, which publishes systematic reviews on health care, by the DoH Health Technology Assessment Programme and others and this information must be fully utilised. In situations where local guidelines need to be produced without the aid of national guidance, managers need to realise their limitations; if they do not know or are uncertain of best practice, they must seek guidance. The ability to critically appraise the strength of evidence available and to apply it should be part of routine practice.

One problem associated with basing decisions on published research is that many studies, for example clinical trials, limit the types of subjects they include and these subjects are often white and middle aged. Recommendations following this work can only then extrapolate to a population similar to the study group, effectively denying access to other groups including ethnic minorities and the elderly. Reasons for this include ignorance, methodological limitations of the research, sampling problems, lack of access to minority communities and language barriers. Reasons for exclusivity need to be cited and once effectiveness has been shown in one group, efforts should be made to roll out research to be more inclusive.

Clinical standards

NSFs will provide a systematic approach to models of service provision by defining service models, setting national standards and putting in place programmes to support implementation. The NICE will be responsible for appraising new interventions, giving guidance on best clinical practice and developing audit methodologies (via the National Centre for Clinical Audit). These clinical standards will help to ensure consistent access to services and quality of care across the country.

The first three NSFs have been published on coronary heart disease, mental health and cancer. All cite ethnic issues; for example, in mental health, the External Reference Group recommended that people with mental health problems should be able to expect that services will:

- involve service users and their carers in planning and delivery of care
- be well suited to those who use them and non-discriminatory
- be well coordinated between all staff and agencies
- be properly accountable to the public, service users and carers.

Risk management

Clinical risk reduction programmes and critical incident reporting have been highlighted in the White Paper *The new NHS: modern, dependable* as main components of clinical governance. Marginal groups are becoming more organised, fuelling the increasing risk of litigation. Clinical risk management aims to achieve four principal objectives:

- proactively to identify areas where failure might occur and remedy them before failure does occur
- reporting incidents when they do occur

Clinical governance

- the subsequent collection of information (for internal investigation, facilitating a speedy settlement or allowing those involved to learn from their experience)
- if all else fails, adequate information will be available for future defence in litigation.

Monitoring and evaluation

Scrutiny will occur both internally (professional self-regulation, audit) and externally (CHI, the National Survey of Patient and User Experiences). The National Performance Assessment Framework has provided the six key areas in which standards should be set and measured: health improvement, fair access, effectiveness, efficiency, patient and carer experiences and health outcome of NHS care. The increasing involvement of patients and carers in the monitoring and evaluation of patient care is seen by many health care workers as threatening. However, this group, so intimately involved, give very personal views of the health care system 'from the other side', something health care workers themselves are unable to do. Their opinions on health care may be widely different from the more traditional opinions given by doctors and nurses, but equally valid. The new NSF on mental health emphasises that service users and their carers should be involved in the planning and delivery of care.

National Confidential Inquiries

The four existing National Confidential Inquiries (into perioperative deaths, stillbirths and deaths in infancy, maternal deaths and suicides) will continue but will be overseen by the NICE.

Job plan and individual performance

Appraisal of individual performance is key to improving standards and ensuring individual needs are being met. The job plan will form the basic structure of appraisal and will highlight any areas within the job that are not being met, both currently and as the job develops. Integral to the job plan is continuing professional development, essential for maintaining and developing professional knowledge and competence. This is discussed below. Assessment of individual performance should be facilitative and explore issues of diversity in access; for example, the needs of overseas nurses and language skills.

Diversity and service quality

Continuing professional development

This is about developing a culture that encourages lifelong learning (the learning organisation) and is an integral part of the job plan. It enables individuals to maximise their potential, as important to improving patient care as it is to managing diversity. Part-time workers often have poorer access to training facilities, of particular importance to nursing staff. Both internal and external peer review will be an important tool for assessing the effectiveness of the clinical governance culture and in creating a facilitative environment in which excellence can flourish.

Complaints

Complaints will be monitored both externally and internally. There will have to be an effective local system in place to deal with complaints. Documentation will be essential in order to facilitate external scrutiny. It is particularly important that the complaints procedure is made accessible to non-English speakers and to the visually impaired, two groups of patients that may find it very difficult to know how to make themselves heard.

Manpower planning

This will establish the required staffing levels to achieve acceptable standards of care. However, this is not just about recruiting the appropriate staff but also about retaining them. Patients come from all walks of life and managers need to be aware of this when appointing staff.

Whistle blowing

This is to be encouraged. If badly performing work colleagues are not dealt with or reported, responsibility will be shared. This balance between collective and individual responsibility is very important and must be appreciated. Racism and other forms of discrimination should be informed on.

Figure 12.1 summarises the key components (tools) of the clinical governance system and the close link between these tools and Table 12.1 summarises where each component fits in to the evaluation programme.

Clinical governance

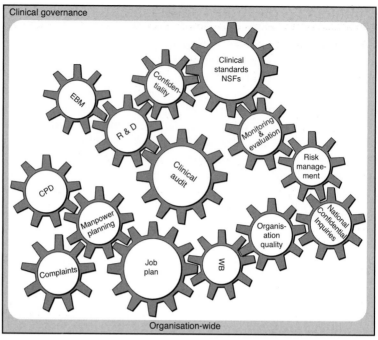

Figure 12.1 The system of clinical governance and its components (tools)
© (reproduced with permission from the Royal Society of Medicine, London)

Table 12.1 Tools available to set (identify), apply and monitor standards

Set (identify)	Apply	Monitor
Evidence-based medicine	Manpower planning	Clinical audit
Clinical standards	CPD and lifelong learning	National inquiries
Research and development	Job plan	Complaints monitoring and evaluation
	Risk management	Whistle blowing

CONCLUSION

Clinical governance is a framework for the improvement of patient care through commitment to high standards, reflective practice, risk management and personal and team development and aims to

> **Box 12.2** The main components (tools) of clinical governance
>
> **The ten key components**
> 1. Clinical audit (individual and service)
> 2. National Confidential Inquiries (e.g. CEPOD)
> 3. Evidence-based medicine (?apply into practice)
> 4. Clinical standards (NSFs, NICE, local)
> 5. Manpower planning (including retention)
> 6. CPD and lifelong learning
> 7. Confidentiality (Caldicot)
> 8. Outcome measures (clinical care: individual and service performance)
> 9. Research and development (including evaluation of care)
> 10. Clinical care quality integrated with organisational quality
>
> **Other components**
> 11. Clinical risk (self and programme(s))
> 12. Complaints
> 13. Job plan and individual performance
> 14. Critical appraisal
> 15. Whistle blowing

put high-quality care at the heart of all decisions made, at whatever level, within the NHS. In order to put it high on the agenda for all NHS staff, the government has specified a number of statutory requirements and for the first time has put clinical governance alongside financial responsibility.

Management can contribute greatly to the success of clinical governance by harnessing and embracing the very different subcultures that work within the NHS and realising that different attitudes and approaches can be good for the organisation. It is important to ensure that these different groups do not feel threatened by differences of approach or opinion and that they are willing and able to work together. Finally, they need to ensure that those accessing care are not discriminated against.

Discussion questions

- In relation to diversity and inequality, reflect on how you might apply the clinical governance framework to contribute to the improvement and maintenance of quality in your own service.
- Which tools do you see as most essential in this and why?

Clinical governance

References

Chief Medical Officer 1999 Clinical governance. Department of Health, London

Donald A 2000 Becoming the future: changing clinical behaviour. In: Rawaf S, Orton P (eds) Health improvement programmes. Royal Society of Medicine, London

Secretary of State for Health 1997 The new NHS: modern, dependable. Stationery Office, London

Diversity and service quality

Application 12:1

Sam Ayer

The care of dependent people: applying the standards matrix

INTRODUCTION

The common experience of vulnerable people is that they are dependent on others to meet their health, social care and financial needs. As nurses working with vulnerable clients such as people with mental health problems and those with learning disabilities, our overall duties are to maintain public trust and confidence in our ability to provide safe and effective care for clients.

One way of meeting these requirements is through professional development which will enhance our awareness and understanding of our own professional accountability by helping to think through courses of action in relation to particular ethical and professional issues. For example, a key role of nurses is to speak up for their clients and act as advocates. Obtaining informed consent from their client before they give any treatment or care is also an important responsibility. For detailed discussions relating to the exercise of professional judgement when working with vulnerable clients, see UKCC 1992a, b, 1996.

THE STANDARDS MATRIX

A well-recognised tool for setting standards for the care of vulnerable individuals by health care practitioners is the standards matrix, developed by the All-Wales Nurse Manpower Committee to examine the current life experience of people with learning disabilities (Welsh Office 1988). The matrix identifies specific service aims to ensure that the special needs of this client group are appropriately considered and met and that their basic human rights are not compromised. It is also ideal for reviewing any type of human services provided for vulnerable groups in society such as in

303

the care of elderly people, people with mental health problems and those who are physically disabled.

The matrix (Fig. 12.1.1) identifies seven key elements, which provide a structure for the analysis of the individual's quality of life.

	Residence	Occupation	Leisure
Community presence Everyone should be within ordinary communities and using facilities available in the same locality	1 Everyone should live in an ordinary house/flat within natural centres of population	2 Working days should be spent in centres of learning, e.g. schools, colleges or places of work, e.g. office, shop, factory, alongside non-handicapped people	3 Regular use should be made of public amenities, e.g. cinemas, restaurants, swimming pool, leisure centres, alongside non-handicapped people
Competence Everyone should be given the opportunity to learn and grow and experience increasing capability	4 The home should be used as a place where domestic skills are gained. It may also be used as a base from which other skills are acquired	5 The working day should be a time for acquiring academic or work-based skills, including job-finding skills	6 Leisure time should be used in acquiring the ability to participate and pursue activities and interests, e.g. sport and hobbies
Choice Everyone should be offered choices and supported and informed in making both major life and day-to-day decisions	7 Everyone should be supported in making major decisions, e.g. where to live, and day-to-day decisions, e.g. when to rise, when to bath. Also it should be ensured that basic human rights are safeguarded	8 A range of meaningful day occupations must be available, i.e. paid employment, further education. For most adults, their income arises from their daytime occupation	9 People should be supported in expressing their personal interests by choosing from a range of activities
Individuality Recognition of the uniqueness of each person and ensuring that opportunities exist for individual self-expression	10 An individual's home should reflect their own personal identity in terms of decoration, effects, etc.	11 Skills and interests of an individual should be matched to their occupation	12 Activities undertaken should express the individual's personal interests
Status and respect Each individual should be encouraged to present themselves in a way that promotes their own self-esteem	13 A person's home and their appearance must enhance their image as citizens within an ordinary community	14 The activities undertaken by individuals and the settings in which they take place should reflect their age and portray them as contributing members of their community	15 The way in which people spend their leisure time should positively enhance their position in society, e.g. type of activity, time it takes place, equipment used, with whom they participate
Continuity Each individual should experience a natural progression in their lives. Where a change occurs in one area of life, care should be taken to minimise disruption in others	16 With growing age, people should progress towards a home of their own. When people move, possessions and relationships should remain familiar	17 People should progress naturally from school to training to work. Any change of occupation should be in line with increased expectations	18 Leisure activities can provide a focus for continuity in people's lives. Where changes occur in other areas of life, familiar activities will act as a link between previous and new situations
Relationships/ partnerships Everyone should be a part of a community with a network of friends and family. Some of these relationships will have deeper attachments	19 People's homes should provide the focus for some of the closest relationships. It will also be a basis for other relationships, e.g. neighbours and the wider community	20 A person's workplace will offer opportunities for further relationships. e.g. colleagues, workmates, trainers, teachers, managers, employers	21 The development of relationships should be an aspect of leisure activities and be undertaken with friends and associates of the individual's own choosing

Figure 12.1.1   Standards matrix

These have been crossreferenced with the three major elements of their day; that is, where people live, how they occupy themselves and how they spend their leisure time.

USING THE STANDARDS MATRIX

The matrix can be used by care managers to carry out a broad examination of the overall service provided to groups of clients. It can also be applied to a review of services to individual clients. In using this matrix, the practitioner will need to think of the relevant questions with which to guide the assessment of standards of care. Some reflective questions are as follows.

Place of residence

- Did the group choose where they now live and who to live with?
- What use is made of local facilities such as shops, transport and cinema?
- In what ways are the client group involved in the running of where they live?
- Do they own their personal belongings, clothing and furniture?
- Are the design, facilities, possessions and clothing age-appropriate?
- Who are involved in clients' care?
- Are staff duties planned to ensure continuity?
- How is family contact maintained?
- What relationships have the group developed?

Daytime occupation

- How is the group occupied regularly during the standard waking day?
- Are the clients provided with the opportunity to learn and earn?
- Is the occupation age-appropriate?
- Is there a distinction between carers and staff support in workplaces?

Use of leisure

- Do the clients use generic facilities?
- Is there a range of leisure activities?
- Can clients afford activity of their choice?
- Have clients' interests been identified?
- Is the timing of and type of activity age-appropriate?

The care of dependent people

Six Steps to **Effective Management**

- If a change of residence occurs is there a continuum of activity for clients?
- Do clients choose with whom they spend their leisure hours?

References

United Kingdom Central Council 1992a Code of professional conduct, UKCC, London

United Kingdom Central Council 1992b The scope of professional practice. UKCC, London

United Kingdom Central Council 1996 Guidelines for mental health and learning disabilities nursing. UKCC, London

Welsh Office 1988 Standards matrix: residential services for mentally handicapped people. Welsh Office, Cardiff

Diversity and service quality

Application 12:2
Louisa Baxter

An occupation, not a characterisation: meeting the health care needs of drug-using prostitutes

INTRODUCTION

Female prostitution is one end of a spectrum of occupations which many women in the face of both gender and economic inequalities can engage in. However, the stigma associated with the selling of sex has tended to turn a socioeconomic issue into one of morality, women who engage in prostitution being generally regarded as deviants and heavily stigmatised (Delmont 1980). The illegality and covert nature of prostitution serves to compound the marginalisation of this group of women, creating barriers to their access to health and social care.

Although they are a heterogeneous group, prostitutes have health needs specific to their occupation, alongside needs resulting from poverty and gender. They work from differing occupational settings in escort services, brothels, 'saunas' and on the streets. Street prostitutes are, however, particularly vulnerable since they tend to be poorer and have less control over the environment in which they work. Furthermore, their pattern of working often involves a chaotic lifestyle, which makes maintaining contact with health services difficult.

In this chapter, a hypothetical case brings together a number of issues to open up a discourse on the health needs of female street prostitutes from the perspective of an outreach worker in a targeted outreach nighttime centre. It concludes with suggestions for improving access to services for this client group.

An occupation, not a characterisation

307

Case study 12.2.1   Marie

Marie is a 24-year-old white woman living in council accommodation in the Manchester area and has worked as a prostitute for 5 years. She began using drugs when she was 16, is now an intravenous drug user with a heroin habit costing £100 a day and reports secondary use of amphetamines, crack cocaine, ecstasy, marijuana and alcohol. Marie also reports sharing injecting equipment 'a few times' in the last 6 months with 'a mate from the beat' and her partner. Marie is also a smoker. She has a 3-year-old daughter whom she cares for with the help of her mother. Marie entered into prostitution to help pay for her drugs but notes an escalation in her drug use as a result.

She sees between two and 10 clients a night and offers full intercourse, oral sex and 'hand relief'. She attempts to always use a condom but reports incidences of unprotected sex for the 'right price', with regulars or when she has been very intoxicated. Marie has been raped twice in the past year and has reported one of these assaults to the police. The man was never caught.

Marie has had her first hepatitis B vaccination at an outreach centre but missed her second. She reports a good general level of health but suffers from tooth decay, occasional abscesses and chest infections. She uses the outreach centre primarily for the needle exchange service but also for free condoms and as a 'safe space' on the streets.

PROSTITUTES' HEALTH CARE NEEDS

Violence

Violence has been identified as a leading cause of concern for the health of prostitutes (Faugier et al 1997). This can take the form of muggings, rape and physical violence directed at the women by clients, other prostitutes, partners, the general public and the police. These attacks are rarely reported due to a desire for self-sufficiency and/or fear that the various authorities will not take them seriously. Furthermore, prostitutes can often feel obliged to grant sexual favours to the police in return for immunity from prosecution. In many cases, women do not feel that they can rely on the police for protection from crime.

Some form of violent assault is often the trigger for the first contact that a prostitute may have with mainstream health services for treatment in A & E departments or by a police surgeon. The psychological trauma which may develop after chronic exposure to violence can be profound. Alongside the implications for personal safety, violence reinforces the stigma and further isolates them from mainstream health and social support.

Diversity and service quality

Substance misuse

The long-standing association between prostitution and drug use has been widely documented (see, for example, Goldstein 1979, Darrow 1990). Current research suggests that in some areas intravenous drug use amongst prostitutes is as high as 70% and 60% of intravenous drug users use prostitution to fund an existing habit (MASH 1997). Involvement in prostitution may lead to escalation in drug use and this is linked to greater occupational risk behaviour: for example, longer hours spent working on the street and involvement in higher risk sexual activity. Drug-using women are the more vulnerable group of prostitutes on the street. They face more exploitation by customers, are less able to negotiate within the client/prostitute transaction and have less control over themselves or their environment.

Intravenous drug users also report higher general levels of injury and infection, including hepatitis B and C. Their health needs may be secondary to procuring adequate funds for drugs. Fear of legal reprisals for their drug use and their often chaotic lifestyle may mean that they are less likely to initiate or maintain contact with mainstream services.

Sexual health

Sexual health is indicated as another leading cause of concern in relation to this client group, contraction of sexually transmitted diseases, in particular HIV, being one of the main occupational health hazards. As a result of aggressive health education campaigns over the last decade, however, women are increasingly becoming aware of the health risks and the necessity to take precautions to safeguard their health and that of their clients. This is reflected by work carried out by Carr (1995). Intravenous drug users, however, may have lower levels of condom use and may be targeted by customers for higher risk sexual activities.

It is significant that it was the rising number of HIV and AIDS cases in the general Western population in the early 1990s which thrust prostitution into the forefront of government resources and policy, female prostitutes being blamed for the explosion of the disease (Carr 1995). Whilst any diversion of resources to an underresourced group is welcome, viewing prostitutes primarily as 'reservoirs of infection' has engendered a situation whereby health professionals tend to approach them primarily from the perspective of safer professional sex. From the author's own experience of outreach work with prostitutes, it is evident that some resent the health professionals' overemphasis on safe sex information which they feel is often provided at the expense of attention to their own expressed health needs.

The legal, moral and ethical debates that surround the occupation often tend to portray prostitutes as solely responsible for sexual

An occupation, not a characterisation

behaviour within the client/prostitute transaction; dialogue about the men involved is all too often absent in discourse on this industry. Work by Faugier et al (1997) provides strong evidence that increased risk-taking behaviour on the part of female prostitutes is more strongly associated with economic necessity and it is the 'punters' who will instigate more risky behaviour within the transaction. The authors argue, therefore, that this group of men should equally be the focus of such health education messages (Faugier & Cranfeild 1997).

Mental illness

A study of the profiles of some prostitutes indicates that many have suffered from social and/or economic deprivation as a child. This may include emotional, sexual or psychological abuse, being placed in care as a child, leaving school before the required age, drug use beginning at an early age, a teenage pregnancy or abortion. Such experiences of deprivation and loss may be triggers for mental illness (Davidson 1999, Green 1992, Linehan 1997, Silverman et al 1996).

This has profound implications for the knowledge, skills, awareness and attitudes of care providers who work with children in care homes, with young offenders or children on childcare registers. Faugier & Sargeant (1997) emphasise that strategies for improving the self-esteem of children in these situations and to empower them to make healthy choices and to find other avenues through which to support themselves and their families are thus a vital part of childcare services.

Negative attitudes and prejudice

Some prostitutes report negative reactions when they disclose their occupation to health care professionals. Such reactions act as a barrier to seeking assistance, to maintaining contact with and to full disclosure to service providers. This can lead to poor uptake of services and treatment specific to their health concerns. The tendency amongst prostitutes to withhold information about socially unacceptable behaviours and activities from nurses and doctors stems from a fear of legal reprisals, in particular losing custody of their children. This may be compounded by the fact that there may be reluctance among general practitioners to take on prostitutes as patients, either for financial or moral reasons (Lipley 1999).

However, prostitutes, feel that they are not always able to rely on service providers to afford them confidentiality and to provide them with a network of support in which women are encouraged to keep their children. This profound mistrust of health professionals by prostitutes must be recognised. Faugier et al (1997) report that, of the 118 women registered with a general practitioner, the majority (86) said they did not tell the doctor what they did and only 22 of the 73 who had a drug habit revealed this to the doctor. Even more disconcerting is that the majority of women said the GP did not ask their occupation, even when they presented with a genitourinary problem.

There is now a strong lobby to bring about reforms in relation to the law and prostitution. At the instigation of the RCN, groups with an interest in the impact of prostitution met and agreed that prostitutes should have easy access to primary care, be able to disclose their occupation to health care professionals and should not be the victims of prejudice when they are being treated. The RCN Congress has also backed a resolution calling for the decriminalisation of the occupation and for new laws which allow prostitutes to work in small groups from their own premises without a licence and allow licensing for larger commercial establishments (Nursing Standard 1995, 1996).

Decriminalisation has traditionally been cited as a solution to the problems of prostitutes having to work in covert ways and thus becoming isolated from health and social services. The real issue, however, is that changing attitudes to female sexuality and the status of women is as vital as the socioeconomic reforms that protect and affirm them. Only this will ensure that women 'choose' to work as prostitutes and that those who do so work in an environment that is regulated to minimise their exploitation and ensure their safety.

IMPROVING ACCESS TO HEALTH CARE

Prostitution is an occupation, not a characterisation, a factor which should be borne in mind by all those providing care and support.

Within mainstream services, there is an urgent requirement to carry out assessment of these women's needs and, where appropriate, refer to specialist services. Prostitutes, however, feel better able to use services which they see as user friendly, appropriate and relevant to their needs, where they are not likely to be treated in a judgemental manner and are guaranteed confidentiality. Nurses are often at the frontline of care. As facilitators of health care, they are important avenues by which positive attitudes to prostitutes' health may be promoted.

Nurse managers are required to promote standards of good practice in this area, paying attention to ensuring easier access to the relevant services by removing the barriers enforced by judgemental attitudes. They will be responsible for ensuring that staff have the specialist training and support required in managing people with drug problems and discussing sexual issues.

Siting general health care at drug and genitourinary medical services may lead to greater uptake generally but many women do not currently use these services or see them as relevant to their needs and lifestyles (Faugier et al 1997). The peripatetic lifestyle of street prostitutes requires services to be flexible and available at the times when they are likely to use them.

An occupation, not a characterisation

Six Steps to **Effective Management**

Targeted outreach delivered by non-governmental organisations plays a very important role in providing practical support and health care. Common features of these services are:

- support and care from both a health and service perspective
- multidisciplinary staff mix with a core of nursing and other health and social care staff (the effectiveness of this approach in preventing the spread of HIV infection has been evidenced in work carried out in Glasgow (Carr et al 1996))
- mobile nighttime unit which takes the service to where the women are – this could be used for delivering hepatitis B vaccination programmes and screening for hepatitis C disease
- practical assistance with meeting basic needs such as shelter, housing, childcare and access to benefits.

References

Carr S V 1995 The health of women working in the sex industry: a moral and ethical perspective. Sexual and Marital Therapy 10(2):201–213

Carr S V, Goldberg D J, Elliot Green S, Machu C, Cruer L 1996 In practice: a primary health care service for Glasgow street sex workers: six years of experience of drop in centre, 1989–1994. AIDS Care 8(4):489–497

Darrow W W 1990 Prostitution, intravenous drug use, and HIV-1 in the United States. In: Plant M (ed) AIDS, drugs and prostitution. Routledge, London, pp 18–41

Davidson L 1999 School age prostitution: an issue for children's nurses? Journal of Child Health Care 3(2):5–10

Delmont S 1980 Sociology of women. Allen and Unwin, London

Faugier J, Cranfeild S 1997 Reaching male clients of female prostitutes: the challenge for HIV prevention. AIDS Care 1 (suppl):S21–S32

Faugier J, Sargeant M 1997 Positive awareness: health professionals' response to child protection. In: Barrett D (ed) Child protection in Britain. The Children Society, London

Faugier J, Cranfeild S, Sargeant M 1997 Risk behaviors and healthcare needs of drug using female prostitutes. Journal of Substance Abuse 2:203–209

Goldstein P J 1979 Prostitution and drugs. Lexington, New York

Green J 1992 It's no game. National Youth Agency, Leicester

Linehan T 1997 Insight, who cares: child prostitution. Nursing Times 93(22):22–25

Lipley N 1999 Street life. Nursing Standard 13 (48):18–24

Manchester Action on Street Health 1997 Annual report. MASH, Manchester

Nursing Standard 1995 News: council seeks better care access for prostitutes. Nursing Standard 10(5)

Nursing Standard 1996 News: prostitutes' rights to equal treatment. Nursing Standard 10(21)

Silverman A B, Reinherz H Z, Giaconia R M 1996 The long-term sequelae of child and adolescent abuse. A longitudinal community study. Child Abuse and Neglect 20(8):709–723

Diversity and service quality

Application **12:3**

Carol Baxter, Peter Toon

The nursing care of lesbians and gay men

INTRODUCTION

This chapter has three elements:

- an RCN statement on the nursing care of lesbians and gay men
- three complex cases, based on real-life experiences involving the nursing care of lesbians or gay men
- commentaries on these cases, indicating the issues that need to be considered by the nurse manager in addressing each one.

Read the RCN statement and then read each case, slowly and thoughtfully. Imagine yourself in the position of the nurse in each case. Visualise the scene, listen to the sound of the voices, imagine the conversations. How does it make you feel?

Reflect on how you would handle each situation if you were the responsible manager, bearing in mind the RCN's statement on the nursing care of gay and lesbian patients.

THE NURSING CARE OF LELBIANS AND GAY MEN: AN RCN STATEMENT

The RCN recognises through work undertaken by its members that discrimination and prejudice towards lesbian and gay patients exist in nursing.

This statement outlines the RCN's commitment to developing and promoting good nursing practice for this group of clients and to the support and assistance of any nurses who experience difficulties in developing their practice in this area.

Six Steps to **Effective Management**

What are the actual and potential unmet nursing needs of lesbians and gay men?

There is now a growing body of literature exploring the health care needs and experiences of lesbians and gay men. The literature demonstrates that people in this client group are exposed to many specific and additional stresses as users of the health service (Platzer 1993).

- They have concerns that relate to homophobia or anti-lesbian and gay feelings from doctors and health care providers in general.
- Some lesbian and gay patients fear the consequences of being open about their sexuality but also believe they cannot always get the relevant care they need if they are not open.
- Some people fear that they may even be physically harmed if health care practitioners are homophobic and/or that a breach of confidentiality could have negative consequences for them in relation to employment, housing, child custody or future health care.

Lesbian and gay patients report experiencing negative and hostile reactions from health care practitioners when their sexual orientation is known. It has also been found that negative reactions, or even fear of such reactions, may prevent lesbians and gay men from seeking health care when it is needed.

In addition to this, the literature suggests that lesbians and gay men have particular health needs which nurses should be aware of. The pressures of living as a lesbian or gay man in a society which has intense negative and condemning taboos against them may have consequences for their physical and mental health.

- There is evidence of a much higher incidence of alcohol abuse in the lesbian and gay population which may be related to such stress.
- There is also evidence that lesbian and gay teenagers are particularly at risk from mental and physical health problems. This is due to the lack of support they receive when trying to come to terms with their difference from accepted social norms. The high attempted suicide rate in this group is an indication of the importance which should be attached to addressing their health care needs and raising awareness amongst nurses of such needs.
- There are suggestions that there are many other areas, as yet unresearched, in which the health status of lesbians and gay men is prejudiced; nurses need to explore these.

Diversity and service quality

How can nurses address these concerns?

It is clear that lesbians and gay men have specific health care needs and concerns which nurses probably do not address. A concerted response is required from the profession if we are to fulfil the collective and individual responsibilities implied by the UKCC *Code of professional conduct* in relation to this client group.

- *Nurses in clinical practice* need to ensure that they never intentionally behave in a way which marginalises this client group. They must: examine their behaviour towards clients to ensure that it cannot be considered as prejudicial; actively seek to raise awareness of the problem amongst colleagues; discourage unhelpful responses and explore all possible ways of supporting and assisting lesbians and gay men using their service.
- *Nurses undertaking research* need to develop studies of lesbians' and gay men's actual and perceived health care experiences and should establish how they can best meet the needs of their lesbian and gay patients.
- *Nurses in education* need to recognise the need for the profession to be better informed and to have more positive attitudes in these areas and to design pre- and postregistration training and education strategies that recognise this.
- *Nurses in purchasing* need to recognise the potential of the nursing contribution towards health gain for this client group and to reflect this in the contract specification agreed with providers.
- *Nurses in management* need to promote good practice in this area and ensure that equal opportunities in relation to service provision are adequately addressed.

Nurses also need to challenge homophobia and prejudice in the workplace wherever they encounter it.

Advice and assistance from the RCN

The RCN will continue to support the development of robust nursing practice in this area by supporting the Lesbian and Gay Nursing Needs Working Party and promoting its work. Any member who requires advice and assistance from the RCN in relation to their own practice can contact the working group via their regional office or through the Department of Nursing Policy and Practice at Headquarters (0207 872 0840).

Nursing care of lesbians and gay men

CASE STUDIES

Case study 12.3.1

You are working as a nurse on a hospice ward. You are the named nurse for Andrew, a 32-year-old gay man with advanced HIV infection with a number of complications. He is not expected to live more than a few weeks. James, his boyfriend, visits daily and spends every evening on the ward. They have been together for 5 years and Simon has named James as next of kin in his nursing notes. A number of other gay friends also visit frequently.

One weekend Andrew's parents, who live some distance away but phone daily, arrive. They want to discuss arrangements for Andrew to 'come home', as they put it, with them. They have discussed this with their local hospice, which has a home care support team who are happy to provide nursing support, and their GP who has known Andrew since he was a child and is keen to help.

Andrew is clearly unhappy about the proposal but equally clearly does not wish to upset them. You can see that though he says very little, James meanwhile is seething with rage.

Case study 12.3.2

You are a practice nurse in a baby clinic, doing the immunisations. A woman whom you don't know brings a 12-month-old baby, on your list as Giles Harwood, for MMR. When you greet her as Ms Harwood she replies 'Oh no, I'm not Elaine Harwood, she's my partner, I'm Jane Derby'.

You proceed to explain the immunisation and mention concerns arising from the recent controversy. She comments 'Oh yes, we've been into all that. Sean, the baby's father, isn't very keen for him to have it, but Elaine and I have talked it through and we are sure that it is the right thing to do'.

Case study 12.3.3

You are a nurse working in a health promotion unit. Your health authority has been running an advice line and free condom distribution service via the gay clubs in your town. You overhear the head of the Public Health Department, discussing future plans with the Chair of the PCG, say 'I think it's about time we stopped subsidising the queers' sex games, don't you?'. You find this particularly offensive, since you are gay yourself.

Diversity and service quality

Imagine yourself in the position of the nurse in each case. Visualise the scene, listen to the sound of the voices, imagine the conversations. How does it make you feel?

Reflect on how you would handle each situation, bearing in mind the RCN's statement on the nursing care of gay and lesbian patients.

ISSUES AND STRATEGIES

Case study 12.3.1

Although you will naturally try to do your best for all parties in this situation, the needs and desires of your patient must be paramount. He has clearly expressed these wishes by naming James and not his parents as the next of kin. How can this best be made clear to his parents and how can he be encouraged and supported in making his true feelings known?

Even when they are apparently accepting of a gay relationship, many heterosexuals subconsciously consider them to be less 'real' or important than heterosexual ones (as in the notorious Section 28 phrase 'pretended family relationships'). This can be very hurtful to gay people whose deepest feelings are thus devalued, particularly when facing the imminent or recent death of a lifelong partner. Imagine the situation if Andrew were heterosexual and it was not James but Jemima, his wife?

Although they may have acted precipitately, Andrew's parents no doubt have the best of motives. How can they and all those whom they have mobilised best be made to accept that their careful plans may not be what the patient wants?

As the nurse or nurse manager, how do you resist social pressures to conform and to compromise what you believe in? Does the RCN statement help you in this respect?

Case study 12.3.2

Again, there is the problem of how you acknowledge the validity of a relationship which is important and real to those involved, however unconventional it may be. Here you face the additional problem that whatever Jane and Elaine have decided between them, the legal situation may well be more complex. Is Jane legally appointed as Giles' guardian? If not, then strictly she has no right to consent to the immunisation. What is Sean's position? Has he voluntarily abandoned his parental rights and duties? To act on the instruction of one parent when you know that the other opposes your action is asking for litigation.

How can you explore these complexities without making Jane feel insulted that you do not think that she is the baby's real parent?

Six Steps to **Effective Management**

What procedures and guidelines on parental consent exist in your health authority that would help you to deal with this (and other extramarital, non-traditional relationships)?

Case study 12.3.3

This case raises two issues:

- homophobia in the workplace as it affects gay and lesbian staff
- homophobic influences on public health priorities.

Many gay and lesbian health workers feel insecure about being open about their sexuality at work, for fear of discrimination and victimisation. How as a manager can you create an environment where gay and lesbian staff can feel secure that they will not be discriminated against on the grounds of their sexuality? How do you tackle such homophobic remarks and the attitudes which underlie them in a way which both acknowledges the unacceptability of homophobic attitudes and at the same time improves relationships between gay and heterosexual staff rather than promotes tension?

Public health priorities should be set according to need and discrimination on grounds of race, religion, sexuality, or any other social characteristic, should be unacceptable. But this is easier said than done. How would you set about evaluating your anti-HIV strategy against other priorities in a way that would not discriminate on grounds of sexuality?

Further reading

Akinsanya J, Rouse P 1991 Who will care? A survey of the knowledge and attitudes of hospital nurses towards people with HIV/AIDS. Department of Health, London

Bhugra D, King M 1989 Controlled comparison of attitudes of psychiatrists, general practitioners, homosexual doctors and homosexual men to male homosexuality. Journal of the Royal Society of Medicine 82:603–605

Johnson S R, Palermo J L 1984 Gynaecologic care for lesbian. Clinical Obstetrics and Gynaecology 27(3):724–731

Jones A 1988 Nothing gay about bereavement. Nursing Times 84(23):55–56

Olesker E, Walsh L V 1984 Childbearing among lesbians: are we meeting their needs? Journal of Nurse Midwifery 29(5):322–329

Owen W F 1989 The clinical approach to the male homosexual patient. Medical Clinics of North America 70(3):499–535

Paroski P A 1987 Health care delivery and the concerns of gay and lesbian adolescents. Journal of Adolescent Health Care 8(2):188–192

Royse D, Birge B 1987 Homophobia and attitudes towards AID patients among medical, nursing, and paramedical students. Psychological Reports 61:867–870

Diversity and service quality

Sanford N D 1989 Providing sensitive health care to gay and lesbian youth. Nurse Practitioner 14(5):30–47

Sevens P, Hall E, Srigma J M 1988 Health beliefs and experiences with health care in lesbian women. IMAGE: Journal of Nursing Scholarship 20(2):69–73

Teri L 1982 Effects of sex and sex-role style on clinical judgement. Sex Roles 8(6):636–649

Weeks J 1989 Sex, politics and society: the regulation of sexuality since 1800, 2nd edn. Longman, London

Young E W 1988 Nurses' attitudes toward homosexuality: analysis of change in AIDS workshops. Journal of Continuing Education in Nursing 19(1):9–12

Zeidenstein L 1990 Gynaecologic and childbearing needs of lesbians. Journal of Nurse Midwifery 35(1):10–18

Nursing care of lesbians and gay men

Managing the pain associated with sickle cell disease: learning and leading from evidence-based management practice

INTRODUCTION

Sickle cell disease is an inherited blood disorder. In the UK it primarily affects sections of ethnic minority communities. It has been suggested that this disorder has forced into the health care system ethnic and racial groups who traditionally have experienced less access or acceptability within the health care services (Alleyne & Thomas 1994). The effective management of this condition has continued to challenge health professionals and policy makers, poor management of pain in particular being cited as a major area of concern.

This chapter reflects on the poor experience of patients requiring hospitalisation for pain management and demonstrates how the five Ps (Partnership, Performance, Professions, Patient Care, Prevention) (Jumaa et al 2000) put forward in the government's National Plan for the Health Service can be used as a framework in reversing this trend.

BACKGROUND

Sickle cell disease is an inclusive term for a group of inherited blood disorders which primarily (but not exclusively) affects people of

African, African-Caribbean, Mediterranean, Middle Eastern and Asian ancestry. It is the second highest inherited disorder in Britain today with an estimated 75 children being born with the condition each year. It is a progressive and often disabling illness that can lead to severe clinical consequences, some of which are outlined (in Box 12.4.1).

There is considerable concern regarding the need for improvement in services to people with sickle cell disease (DoH 1993). Undercoverage of the condition in medical and nursing curricula and the need for health professionals to be better informed about this condition, both in terms of a general understanding and about the hands-on clinical care required, are well recognised (DoH 1993, Streetly et al 1993).

There has been a strong perception within the affected community regarding inequalities in the provision of appropriate services for people with sickle cell disease. Over the last 30 years, the community has campaigned for a number of specific areas of service improvement already afforded to other inherited disorders which occur less frequently in the community (Box 12.4.2).

Box 12.4.1 Problems associated with sickle cell disease

Acute problems
- Tiredness, jaundice, slow growth in children and increased susceptibility to infections and painful crises.
- Maternal complications include anaemia, infection, pain, infarction, pulmonary embolism and preeclampsia.
- Pregnancy in women is hazardous to both mother and fetus.
- Fetal risks include early abortion, intrauterine growth retardation, prematurity and stillbirth.

Long-term problems
- Damage to vital organs can result in mechanical disability, renal problems, liver disease and leg ulcers.

Psychological consequences
- Adverse psychological reactions such as lack of maternal and paternal bonding.
- Parental guilt may lead to child abuse and marital discord if its inheritance is not understood.
- This can affect the self-esteem of the black population: feeling of being stigmatised as a consequence of racial link.

Social consequences
- Increased spending on fuel to combat the effect of cold on precipitating crises.
- Schooling and employment can often be interrupted and the lives of the sufferer and his/her family disrupted.

Managing the pain associated with sickle cell disease

> **Box 12.4.2** Services campaigned for by black and ethnic minority communities since the 1970s
>
> - Universal screening for all newborn babies.
> - Preconceptual and antenatal counselling of at-risk couples.
> - Exemption from prescription charges for those suffering from the disease.
> - Recognition of the implications for housing, education and employment.
> - The resourcing and development of specialist centres for treatment and practical support in the community.

A study by Alleyne & Thomas (1994) concluded that one of the damaging consequences in the context of sickle cell care is the level of neglect and dissatisfaction that the service users experience, with the perception that healthcare staff are often being alienated from the patients. This is expressed through hostile and uncaring attitudes and behaviour.

PAIN IN SICKLE CELL DISEASE: THE HIGH COST OF DOUBT

The disease is characterised by a defective haemoglobin molecule (HbS) which, under certain conditions, causes the red blood cell to become sickle (crescent) shaped. This causes impaired circulation, inadequate oxygenation, pain and tissue infarction, resulting in damage to vital organs. The pain (commonly called crisis) occurs when misshapen blood cells create capillary blockages and is episodic and severe, often requiring repeated hospitalisation for pain management for some individuals. Periodic episodes of pain can occur in the arms and legs, back, abdomen or chest over a prolonged period, the occurrence and severity varying from person to person. The degree of pain experienced during a crisis has been compared to that of another form of infarct, myocardial infarction. Patients with evolving myocardial infarction typically receive immediate and aggressive treatment from health care personnel to prevent further cardiac damage; those in pain from sickle cell crisis do not receive anything like the same attention (Gorman 1999).

Research has consistently demonstrated that patients' experiences of hospital care during a crisis show a range of interrelated themes: stigmatisation, excessive control (including both over- and undertreatment of pain), general neglect and lack of involvement in treatment decisions. In one of the first qualitative studies of this nature in the UK (Alleyne & Thomas 1994), the accounts of all 10 patients interviewed bore testimony to the mismanagement of their painful crises. Patients reported difficulty in obtaining analgesics and of feeling disbelieved. This was reflected in the responses of nurses, such as: 'Are you sure you're due for your medication?' and 'Do you really need it?'.

Such responses were common and verified the patient's perceptions. Reflecting on the level of mistrust which they experienced when requesting painkillers, patients frequently reported resorting to a variety of coping strategies: 'Shout, ring the bell and then shout again'.

Reports of having to wait for unnecessarily long periods to receive medication were also a regular feature of patients' experience: 'You can wait up to half an hour'.

Such delays on the part of nurses to respond to the patient in pain were perceived as deliberate, with nurses misinterpreting the requests for analgesics as 'drug-seeking' behaviour.

> 'I get the feeling that some of them purposely prolong it.'
> 'They don't realise that while they are prolonging it the pain's getting worse and it's stressful.'
> '(The nurses) think that we are two-hour junkies; you know, as soon as the time is up, we want a fix.'

Those nurses who were prepared to speak out on the patients' behalf also confirmed patients' accounts. One nurse who reported witnessing the deliberate 'delaying process' associated with the administration of analgesics to this client group stated:

> The nurse goes huh, walks away, goes into the office, checks the drugs, goes back outside, she really drags her heels, she will do everything to sort of hang on and make the patient wait, and I think that's deliberate.

A similar study carried out more than 5 years later involving 55 patients in London suggests that there has been no change in the experience of this client group (Maxwell et al 1999). The authors state 'that virtually all patients with sickle cell disease were stigmatised as drug addicts – a stereotype which simultaneously feeds on and reinforces the mistrust of patients'. The following quote from a patient interviewed in this qualitative study is significant.

> The nurse turned around to me and said 'It's not because we don't wanna give you the painkillers, it's cos we are scared that you're gonna get hooked on it and we don't wanna see you down on the street hustling drugs.'

In reflecting on an understanding of the history of race relations in the United Kingdom, the authors concluded that their findings:

> ...prompts the question as to what extent do the experiences of mistrust and stigmatisation of patients with sickle cell disease mirror the healthcare experiences of London's black population more generally?

Managing the pain associated with sickle cell disease

Six Steps to **Effective Management**

HOW CAN THIS TREND BE REVERSED? LEARNING AND LEADING FROM EVIDENCE-BASED MANAGEMENT PRACTICE

In seeking to improve the quality and delivery of pain management and care for this client group, service managers will need to appreciate the complex nature of the problem. It is recognised that clinical services are multifaceted and difficult to manage. It is argued that health goals are often ambiguous, roles are not always explicit, processes are often unclear and relationships are not open (Alleyne & Jumaa 1998). The results in this case are distressed and dissatisfied patients and frustrated and angry staff.

Jumaa et al (2000) have proposed an approach to achieve nursing management excellence in such complex situations. This model contends that a radical transformation of existing clinical service models is required and a course of action is described which includes the active involvement and motivation of both staff and patients. This would provide a suitable model in the context of the effective management of painful episodes of sickle cell crisis. Here we will consider how this might be applied to achieve the Five Ps of clinical excellence (Partnership, Performance, Professions, Patient Care, Prevention) in this situation, the challenge being to consider how we are demonstrating our commitment to the following.

Partnership (based on specific goals)

Collaboration with the patient in pain, so that their goal of effective pain relief is achieved. This requires aims of care to be identified which will provide a framework for action and success. The goals can be determined using these criteria, based on the acronym ASTREAM (Achievable, Specific, Time bound, Realistic, Empowered, Agreed, Measurable).

Using this approach requires the nurse to communicate sensitively with the patient, to consider the various options regarding pain relief and to include the patient in the choice of available interventions. A recognition that the 'patient knows best' would be one way in which the patient could be empowered. Another aspect of empowerment is to ensure that the nurse has the resources (THEIMM) to achieve the agreed aims of care.

- *Time (to be with the patient)* – it is the responsibility of the nurse to ensure that this is the case. When this is difficult, either through staff shortage or workload demands, then the nurse must take responsibility and inform the line manager of the situation.
- *Human* – do the staff have the appropriate attitudes, skills and knowledge to effectively manage the care of the patient in pain?

Diversity and service quality

324

- *Equipment* – is there the necessary equipment such as syringe drivers, patient-controlled analgesic pumps, etc. to ensure that the patient receives the medication on time, every time and in a manner which suits them?
- *Information* – do staff have access to and the appropriate skills to implement evidence-based care?
- *Materials* – what other modalities could be utilised to provide effective pain management, such as the use of heat pads or alternative and complementary therapies (rather than total reliance on narcotic analgesics) to provide comfort to the patient?
- *Money* – does the ward budget take account of the numbers and skill mix of staff; for example, to ensure that optimum levels of care are achieved at all times? If there are insufficient funds, who has the ability to make a case for extra funding?

Performance (founded on explicit roles)

In order to achieve clinical effectiveness one has to ask whether the nurses have the knowledge and tools required to assess, plan and implement appropriate interventions and to monitor the severity of pain and the effectiveness of their interventions. This is essential in order to sustain clinical nursing performance.

Professions (performing using clear processes)

How can nurses ensure that they are acting responsibly and are accountable for their actions? What do they need in order to act differently towards the patient in pain? Clear processes are essential to empower nurses to take responsibility for effective pain management. Clinical guidelines are essential for the management. Nurses must accept that mistrust of patients and excessive control over care regimens are not the hallmarks of a professional.

Patient care (within an atmosphere of open relationships)

Creating a 'no blame' culture requires patient involvement in the whole process of care. Acceptance of the patient's expressions of pain and a sensitive, effective response are essential in promoting an open relationship between patient and care provider.

Prevention (of vague goals, implicit goals, unclear processes and a blame culture)

When all of the above has been effectively managed then a 'cultural change' will occur. Empowering nurses and patients, through the

Managing the pain associated with sickle cell disease

Six Steps to **Effective Management**

provision of adequate resources and support structures within the health care organisation, will reduce the climate of conflict, oppression and stress which is currently rife within the context of managing the painful crises of sickle cell disorder.

CONCLUSION

Painful crises are the distinct feature of sickle cell disease both for individual suffering and for service use (Brozovic et al 1987). The mismanagement of pain is a source of much distress for patients with sickle cell disease and of frustration for the staff who care for them. It is recognised that pain is not the only area of care management which needs to be addressed for people with this condition. However, the obvious urgent need for action, coupled with the timely climate of change within the health service, should provide opportunities for the wider challenges in the general management of this condition to be achieved.

References

Alleyne J, Jumaa M O 1998 Using work-based learning methodology to resolve role conflict at work: introducing 'Mansour's matrix'. Paper presented at the 6th International Conference on Experiential Learning, 'Experiential Learning in the context of Lifelong Education', University of Tampere, Finland, 2–5 July

Alleyne J, Thomas V J 1994 The management of sickle cell crisis pain as experienced by patients and their carers. Journal of Advanced Nursing 19: 725–732

Brozovic M, Davis S C, Bromwell A L 1987 Acute admissions of patients with sickle cell disease who live in Britain. British Medical Journal 294:1206–1208

Department of Health 1993 Report on a working party of the Standing Advisory Committee on Sickle Cell, Thalassaemia and Other Haemoglobinopathies. HMSO, London

Gorman K 1999 Sickle cell disease. American Journal of Nursing 99(3)

Jumaa M O, Yaseen T, Shuldham C 2000 The 5 Ps of nursing management. Nursing Management 7(3):6–7

Maxwell K, Streetly A, Bevan D 1999 Experiences of hospital care and treatment seeking for pain from sickle cell disease: qualitative study. British Medical Journal 318:1585–1590

Streetly A, Dick M, Layton M 1993 Sickle cell disease: the case for co-ordinated information. British Medical Journal 306:1491–1492

Diversity and service quality

Application **12:5**

Peter Ryan

The implementation and evaluation of assertive outreach in mental health

INTRODUCTION

An important recent development in mental health service provision has been assertive outreach. This is an approach which emphasises reaching out and engaging proactively with high-risk users in the community, by working in a flexible, responsive and user-centred way in the user's own 'patch'. Assertive outreach has recently received much public attention from the government, mental health users and mental health services themselves. The government has decided to make assertive outreach a central feature of its new mental health policy. Mental health users for their part fear that assertive outreach may affect their civil liberties. Mental health services are themselves under pressure to implement assertive outreach. There is, however, considerable ambiguity around the term itself, about which model is most effective and what skills and resources are required to implement it.

This chapter provides a brief overview of the model of assertive outreach supported most convincingly by the research evidence. It suggests some guidelines for managers for its implementation and proposes that, given the concerns users are expressing about assertive outreach, an important component of its evaluation should be user-centred focused research.

> **Box 12.5.1**   The integration of core skills and psychosocial rehabilitation in assertive community treatment
>
> *Core skills*
> - Engagement
> - Non-office-based community outreach
> - Comprehensive, needs-led assessment
> - Care planning
> - Linkage with community resources (housing, social security, etc.)
> - Maintenance and expansion of social networks
> - Collaboration with inpatient services and prevention of hospitalisation
> - Advocacy
> - Monitoring and review
>
> *Psychosocial rehabilitation skills*
> - Early intervention and symptom management
> - Behavioural family intervention
> - Assistance with daily living and occupational skills

The integration of core skills and psychosocial rehabilitation in assertive community treatment

Perhaps the central feature of the core functions of an assertive outreach team is that it has to be prepared to work on the clients' own territory and to be persistent in trying to contact them in responsive, practical, client-centred ways. It also has to find creative ways of delivering services to people at times and locations that are better suited to people's needs. Assertive outreach is not an office-based service.

In this model, comprehensive need assessment is crucial (Allness & Knoedler 1998). This involves:

- an assessment of client strengths, aspirations and resources, including an account of vocational, educational and social interests
- psychiatric history, status and diagnosis, including assessment of presenting symptomatology, perhaps through systematic assessments such as the Brief Psychiatric Rating Scale (Overall & Gorham 1962)
- housing and living situation
- self-care abilities
- family and social relationships, including assessment of social functioning, perhaps through systematic scales such as the Life Skills Profile (Rosen et al 1989)

Diversity and service quality

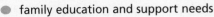
- family education and support needs
- physical health
- alcohol and drug misuse
- an understanding of the gender, ethnic and racial aspects of needs assessment.

Clinical interventions with respect to these core functions include the following.

Direct assistance with meeting basic needs

Staff from the team help clients to meet basic needs for adequate shelter, food and health care in ways that maximise community integration and enhance patient satisfaction. Whenever possible, accommodation is in 'normal' housing rather than specialist mental health housing facilities. Staff visit frequently to assist clients in vivo to develop the appropriate coping skills.

Assistance with a supportive social environment

Staff also focus on assisting patients to develop their own network of family and friends, as well as providing, through their own relationship, a secure source of support. They also run discussion groups and psychoeducational programmes.

Psychosocial rehabilitation skills and functions

A comprehensive series of supporting psychosocial rehabilitation services are offered to the client through the same team.

Early intervention and symptom management

Minimising psychotic symptomatology and the prevention of relapse is given a high priority. Specific interventions include identification of early warning signs and relapse signatures (Birchwood et al 1998), continuous monitoring of appropriate levels of medication, 24-hour crisis availability and occasional brief hospitalisation.

Behavioural family intervention

The team often provides ongoing education to both clients and their families on the nature and management of long-term mental illness. Behavioural family interventions (Fadden 1998) are used in order to optimise communication and support in the family. Essentially this is a form of individually tailored psychoeducational programme which seeks to preserve the family as an asset and resource to the patient. The programme attempts to facilitate a supportive but not

Assertive outreach in mental health

overinvolved or destructive relationship with the patient and the family.

Assistance with daily living and occupational skills

Rather than allocating the client to homogeneous sheltered workshops, the team places great emphasis on developing an individualised occupational plan for each patient. Often this involves part-time work or encouraging a leisure activity. Clients are taught the appropriate occupational skills for the setting and are also supported through any difficulties they might encounter in the work setting. Employers are helped to understand the difficulties the patient may be encountering, are themselves supported through any anxieties or concerns they may be experiencing and are also encouraged to structure the work environment so as to make it more responsive to and accommodating of the client.

AN ACTION FRAMEWORK FOR MANAGERS

Implementing assertive outreach

Critically reflect upon whether you have the following elements of assertive outreach in place.

Team characteristics

- Small caseload (client:team member ratio of 10–15:1).
- Regular review of care plan for each client.
- Team leader is a practitioner with a caseload.
- Continuity of staffing.
- Psychiatrist on staff (client:psychiatrist ratio of 100:1).
- Multidisciplinary staff mix, with a core of nursing, social work and occupational therapy staff, with sessional input from clinical psychology.
- Skill mix includes capability for behavioural/family intervention, early signs monitoring and medication adherence.
- Substance abuse specialist on staff (50:1 ratio).
- Employment rehabilitation specialist on staff (100:1 ratio).
- Community support workers on staff.
- Team consists of at least 10 full-time members.

Organisational boundaries

- Explicit admission criteria.
- Intake rate of six clients per month or fewer.
- Full responsibility for treatment services.

Diversity and service quality

- Responsibility for hospital admission.
- Responsibility for crisis services/24-hour cover.
- Responsibility for hospital discharge planning.
- Service not limited to specific time periods.

User-focused evaluation of assertive outreach

In an important user-controlled study (Beeforth et al 1994) users themselves designed their own evaluation of four assertive outreach teams that had been involved in a major research and development project which had researched the cost and efficacy of these teams (Ryan et al 1999). The authors of the report are themselves service users and are influential members of the UK service user movement. They designed their own semi-structured questionnaire, which explored user perceptions of:

- satisfaction with the service
- their input into and involvement with needs assessment and care planning
- accessibility of the service
- trust and the nature of the client–fieldworker relationship
- their overall quality of life.

Beeforth et al carried out the interviews themselves and also analysed the data and wrote up the report themselves. This was all carried out independently, with no monitoring or control imposed upon them either by the services themselves or by any other professional organisation. In all, 23 service user interviews were conducted across four assertive outreach teams.

Findings

Users were discriminating in their responses and were clear about what they did and did not like and were prepared to say that certain things had improved and certain things had not. They were prepared to say that some things had not worked and this gives increased weight to the positive findings. Nineteen of the 23 users interviewed felt that they had experienced substantial involvement in the needs assessment and care planning process. In terms of accessibility, 15 of the 23 interviewed felt that they were receiving the services they needed, but 10 also felt that they were receiving services they would rather not have. This was largely concerned with dissatisfaction about how medication was dealt with, the inadequate day care services people received and the fact that they sometimes had to go into hospital against their will.

Assertive outreach, as a service in itself, was thought to be different and substantially better than services they normally received with respect to:

Assertive outreach in mental health

Six Steps to **Effective Management**

- accessibility (19 respondents)
- assistance with practical problems (15)
- involvement with the family (8)
- developing community support systems for users (9).

Evaluating assertive outreach from a user perspective

Critically reflect upon the following.

- Do you seriously intend to evaluate assertive outreach from a user perspective? If not, why not?
- Have you identified a group of researcher-users who could coordinate and run this project? Both the Mental Health Foundation (0207 535 7400) and the Sainsbury Centre for Mental Health (0207 403 8790, user-focused monitoring group) work with user researchers.
- Are you prepared to give them freedom to operate?
- At the same time, are you prepared to offer them support and assistance in the project when or if they ask for it?
- Are you prepared to take their results and recommendations seriously and act on them?

References

Allness D J, Knoedler W H 1998 The PACT model of community-based treatment for persons with severe and persistent mental illness: A manual for PACT start-up. NAMI, Virginia

Beeforth M, Conlan E, Grayley R 1994 Have we got views for you. Sainsbury Centre for Mental Health, London

Birchwood M, Todd P, Jackson C 1998 Early intervention in psychosis: the critical period hypothesis. British Journal of Psychiatry 172 (suppl 33):53–59

Fadden G 1998 Family intervention in psychosis. Journal of Mental Health 7(2):115–122

Overall J, Gorham D 1962 The Brief Psychiatric Rating Scale. Psychological Reports 10:799–819

Rosen A, Hadzi-Pavlovic D, Parker G 1989 The Life Skills Profile: a measure assessing function and disability in schizophrenia. Schizophrenia Bulletin 15:325–337

Ryan P, Ford R, Beadsmore A, Muijen M 1999 The enduring relevance of case management. British Journal of Social Work 29:97–125

Further reading

Sainsbury Centre for Mental Health 1998 Keys to engagement: a review of care for people with severe mental illness who are hard to engage with services. Sainsbury Centre for Mental Health, London

Diversity and service quality

Application **12:6**

Carol Baxter, Pauline Ginnety

A comprehensive strategy for the health of Travellers

INTRODUCTION

Travellers are regarded as a distinct ethnic group by the Commission for Racial Equality. The health and health care experience of Travellers is recognised as being worse than that of the mainstream population, poor access to health services being an important component of this. Whereas their traditionally nomadic lifestyle can present challenges to maintaining contact with health services, barriers to access will also result from inflexibility within services and to negative and uninformed attitudes amongst service providers to the travelling culture and way of life.

This chapter briefly describes the work of a project in North Staffordshire Health Authority which is designed to meet the health needs of Travellers, and outlines some questions for managers to reflect on when developing a comprehensive strategy to improve the quality of services to this section of the population.

Box 12.6.1 Improving services for Traveller families: the North Staffordshire Health Authority project

NHS Equality Awards 1998

Local need

This entry for the NHS Equality Awards was made in order to put the issue of Travellers' and gypsies' health needs on the equality agenda in the NHS. The nucleus for early efforts to identify and address the health needs of this population in the country was the Save the Children Fund (SCF) Partnership. This was established in the West Midlands region in 1980 to undertake development work to improve equality of opportunity for Traveller and gypsy families.

333

Diversity and service quality

Box 12.6.1   Cont'd

In 1991 health and social services formed an interagency partnership to address the health needs of Traveller and gypsy families. Since 1996 the primary care manager at NSHA played a leading role in coordinating and directing this work. There are presently three sites in the area, two of which are official, one 'tolerated', and a number of smaller, unofficial (illegal) encampments. A smaller number of Traveller and gypsy families are housed in local authority accommodation.

Equality aims

In terms of the specific health needs of children, a child paediatrician drew attention to the presence of large cases of 'missing underlying pathology', psychological effects of medical problems facing adults and poor connections to other services. Other issues prioritised by members of the group include racial harassment, site needs and conditions, provision of health services and education. Health is considered a primary service, since poor environment and physical health conditions on sites and lack of (or inappropriate) access to local health services negates access by these families to other services, for example social services, housing, police and education specialists (for Traveller and gypsy children in particular).

Further information

The health visitors (one full time and one part time) provide the key day-to-day link between the Traveller and gypsy families and the health agencies. As a result of high levels of illiteracy among Traveller and gypsy families, the health visitors often communicate information about health needs on a one-to-one basis, using word of mouth, pictorial representations and through audiotapes. NSHA has a long-term aim to mainstream provision of health services to Traveller and gypsy families. However, the prevailing culture of ignorance, prejudice, stereotyping and sometimes outright hostility increases the need for continued awareness. The greatest impact made by this project has been the interagency nature of the planning and provision of services to Traveller and gypsy families. Set in the context of the range of needs facing Traveller and gypsy families, the approach taken by the partnership has been to promote the equal opportunities nature of their work. Collectively they have managed to iron out problems of communication between statutory agencies and breakdowns in relationships (as in the past) are increasingly minimised.

(Reproduced with the permission of the Equal Opportunities Unit, NHS Executive, Quarry House, Leeds)

A STRATEGIC APPROACH TO IMPROVING THE QUALITY OF SERVICES TO TRAVELLERS

Basic respect for the nomadic way of life is a prerequisite for competence in meeting the health needs of Travellers. An understanding of the practical implications for the way services are planned and delivered is also essential and services will need to be built on principles of empowerment.

Developing a comprehensive strategy to improve the quality of services to Travellers will require managers to reflect on the following.

- Do your strategic and business plans include a statement on the care of Travellers?
- Are there targets to be met for Travellers in contracts?
- Is there a mechanism for liaising with local councils about information on sites?
- Is there a structured means of communication with A&E units, health centres, local community groups, voluntary agencies and social services departments?
- Is there a flexible approach to cross-boundary work?
- Are policies reviewed to identify discriminatory practices?
- Are Travellers involved in decisions before embarking on initiatives?
- Is there a key worker/designated health visitor appointed to coordinate information and to ensure continuity of care?
- What resources are available for the provision of on-site health care?
- Is the availability of services publicly advertised and made explicit with pictorial aids?
- Are there links between voluntary sector, health and social services?
- Is there a system of patient-held records?
- Are primary care and hospital appointments made to take account of Travellers' lifestyles?

Strategy for the health of Travellers

Index

Index

Index

Index

Index

Six Steps to **Effective Management**

Index